EMBRACING NEURODIVERSITY

with

THE SAFE HOUSE FRAMEWORK

Valli Jones

www.embracingneurodiversity.co/book

For Raymond, you little legend.

Acknowledgements

I want to acknowledge all the people who are doing their bit to improve the state of the world. You know who you are.

To Dad, thank you for getting me to think about how to work differently.

To Rob, thank you for asking thoughtful questions, and for your help with the jobs I don't like doing.

To my kids, thank you for all the sacrifices you have made, knowingly and unknowingly, to make space for my work. I will make it up to you x

CONTENTS

1. BACK STORY

Embracing Neurodiversity is both a personal and professional project. I am a clinical psychologist with a solo private practice on the Gold Coast of Australia, serving mostly neurodivergent folk from early childhood through to about mid-life. I have a particular interest in the internalised presentation of autism, sometimes referred to as the female presentation of autism, though it is evident across genders. I offer diagnostic assessments and therapy, and I have enormous respect and gratitude for the folk who sit with me and work towards self-understanding and, ultimately, some form of inner peace.

The Safe House Framework is the product of years spent observing what helps and what is, at best, unhelpful, and at times, harmful for neurodivergent folk. The framework is a summation of values, knowledge, wisdom, and practical strategies gleaned from sharing time and space with many authentically amazing and unique neurodivergent humans and the wonderful people who love, teach, employ, and care for them. It is an offering for anyone who is neurodivergent, or who knows and /or loves a neurodivergent human.

My intention is to offer a clear and concise blueprint for neurodiversity affirming care, and my hope it that The Safe House Framework will be used as a foundation upon which a kind, respectful, person-centred support system is built for many neurodivergent folk. That is, in a nutshell, the professional aspect of Embracing Neurodiversity.

The personal process of embracing neurodiversity has been less linear and is ongoing. For as long as I can recall, the human mind has fascinated me, so studying psychology as a school-leaver was the natural choice for me. For those who are unfamiliar with the pathways to becoming a psychologist, it is a long and arduous process, and I was nowhere near ready for the post-graduate leg of the journey when I graduated with a bachelor's degree as a young adult. With little thought about where I was headed in my career, I found myself employed in the disability sector, supporting folk in community and residential settings. I also found I had a natural affinity with the autistic people I was supporting, but other than using the insight to guide where I worked, I thought nothing of it. It was not until after I had dipped my toe into a few other potential career options, followed by taking some time out to care for my babies, that I returned to university and registered as a psychologist at the age of thirty-five.

Over the course of a professional deep dive into the internalised presentation of autism, along with a lot of reflection and inward inquiry, and a few painful moments, I have circled around and finally settled into the realisation that I am autistic. On some level I have known since the first time I read a poorly written mainstream media article about 'Invisible Autism' and saw all my personal suffering succinctly expressed in a bullet point list titled 'Characteristic of Asperger's and High Functioning Autism in Females'. There have been countless moments of clarity since, in which I have silently connected the dots of my own experience, occasionally while holding space for another brave soul who is doing the work of self-discovery. My sincere thanks go to those beautiful humans who unknowingly helped me make sense of my internal experience.

I am fortunate to have low support needs, and to have been able to intentionally create a life (a Safe House) for myself that allows me to (mostly) ensure those needs are met. The personal process of embracing neurodiversity continues, and is grounded in self compassion. I choose to believe I am enough, just as I am. To my neurodivergent readers, I hope you also know that you are enough, just as you are. The Safe House is designed to help those who struggle with life in a world set up to cater for a different neurotype, and perhaps doubt their enough-ness.

Note to Readers

'Neurodivergent' is an umbrella term which includes people with a variety of mental and/or behavioural differences, including, but not limited to, autism. I have used the terms 'autistic' and 'neurodivergent' somewhat interchangeably throughout this text. This was a conscious decision, intended to highlight a preference for inclusive language, however I acknowledge that the terms are not interchangeable. Beyond the pages of this book, all autistic people are neurodivergent, but not all neurodivergent people are autistic. Within the pages of this book, the 'Autism Edition', the term neurodivergent refers specifically to autistic people.

2. DESIGNING A SAFE HOUSE

At the time of writing, the dominant cultural narrative is one of autism as a disorder, by definition a cluster of deficits, and broadly considered a difficult problem to be solved. The counter-narrative is one of autism as a reflection of neurodiversity, considered naturally occurring variation within the species, and a valuable piece of humanity. The Safe House Framework occupies the middle ground, leaning heavily towards the latter. Disability is a complex phenomenon, the result of an interaction between biological, psychological, social, and environmental factors. The process of Embracing Neurodiversity involves a shift towards acceptance of differences, a focus on strengths, and a commitment to provision of necessary accommodations and supports. Irrespective of neurotype, humans flourish in accepting, understanding, supportive environments. The Safe House Framework is intended to be a guide for creating spaces for neurodivergent people where the social and environmental barriers to inclusion are addressed to minimise the functional impact of biological factors, and to support psychological wellbeing. In short, it is a framework for neurodiversity affirming care - care that is sensitive to the specific needs and abilities of neurodivergent people, and that reduces the impairment caused by inadequate or inappropriate supports.

In my clinical experience, a diagnosis of autism is almost universally preceded by a period of stress and confusion, and while the diagnosis itself often brings the sort of relief that comes with understanding, the relief is typically accompanied by at least a hint of fear and sadness. Fear about what may lie ahead, and sadness for what may be lost. As the bearer of the news, I feel compelled to reassure parents that their child will be okay. That while the future may look different now, it is still bright. I want to assure them that their child will receive the understanding, care, and acceptance they need to flourish, and because I work in a metropolitan area in a high-income country, I know that some will. However, I also know that the fears of parents are justified. There are a good many children and adolescents who spend too much of their day feeling misunderstood, confused, angry, worried, lonely, or sad. Most of my private practice clients are autistic children and adolescents, and that is how they describe their experience. The stories change, but the emotions are much the same; kids describe the feelings that come with being the square peg, perpetually trying to fit into a round hole. I also sit with people for whom the basic activities of daily living are an enormous challenge and the source of great distress. Despite our country being a place of relative privilege, with socialised health care and a National Disability Insurance Scheme, no one can say with confidence that the services available to autistic folk can or will meet all their needs. The sad reality for many neurodivergent people is that the various systems set up to serve the majority are not suited to them, and engaging with those systems leads to overwhelm, anxiety, depression, and burnout.

The Safe House Framework is a work in progress, and I see it being useful on a few levels. I have structured my thoughts around the image of a house because it captures all the key considerations in a simple visual (neurodivergent minds tend to like visuals):

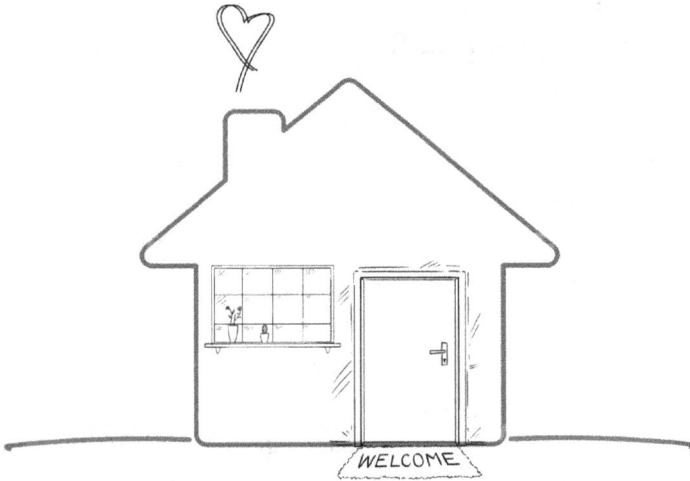

Foundations: the theory, research, and values underpinning neurodiversity affirming care.

Floorplan: the internal experience of autism.

Walls: the intricate human support structure.

Roof: the protective people and systems.

Windows: viewing behaviour as communication of needs.

Door: respectful, authentic connection.

Landscape: the socio-political context.

The tour through the Safe House starts with a brief history of the neurodiversity movement, and a summary of the research supporting a shift from a pathologising model of treatment to a neurodiversity affirming approach to support[1]. This component of the framework provides a context for what follows and applies to all types of neurodivergence. After that, we take a deep dive into the internal experience of autism, the aim of which is to provide a holistic, nuanced understanding of the neurotype, which looks beyond the limited view of autism as defined by the DSM and captures the strengths inherent in the autistic way of being. We then explore the roles and responsibilities of the many people, systems, and structures within an autistic person's life. At an individual level, the framework is essentially a systematic approach to asking questions and gathering information, which in turn allows for a holistic conceptualisation of the neurodivergent person's strengths, differences, and support needs. Foremost, the answers to the questions help to create

---

[1]   I have referred to research literature to highlight avenues for exploration, and I invite those who are interested to peruse the bibliography and read further. My priority has been to keep the content concise, though as someone who is perpetually hyper-focused on topics of interest, I fully appreciate the instinct to dive deep. I have made every effort to compile a thorough list of references for inquisitive minds.

a shared understanding of the neurodivergent person's experience. The answers to the questions also form the basis for the profile of adjustments, accommodations, and supports that will become the Neurodivergent person's Safe House, metaphorically, and in some respects, literally.

On one level, the Safe House Framework is a tool for neurodivergent people and the various people who love, parent, educate, employ, and care for them. It is a framework for organising one's thinking around how best to support neurodivergent folk, and touches on the multitude of external and internal factors which may influence a neurodivergent person's functional capacity, mental health, general wellbeing, and quality of life. The list of factors is by no means exhaustive. However, I have made every effort to take a holistic approach.

On another level, undertaking training in the Safe House Framework offers professionals from any discipline a firm foundation and guide for implementing neurodiversity affirming practices, and a foundation upon which one can refine one's respective professional skill set with the aim of promoting inclusion. Professionals who complete the Masterclass Series will receive Safe House endorsement, and membership of the Safe House Professional Community, an online space where people are invited to connect with like-minded colleagues, and where up-to-date information and resources are shared. Safe House endorsement serves to communicate to neurodivergent service users that a provider or organisation is an informed ally, thus welcoming and facilitating open, honest, and helpful conversations. The aim is not for helping professionals to have all the answers. Rather, endorsement denotes a standard of knowledge around the neurodiversity affirming approach, and signals a commitment to inclusive, respectful, affirming practices. The aim, therefore, is for helping professionals to ask the right questions, creating a context within which neurodivergent folk are supported to self-advocate. The Safe House is emblematic of the felt sense of safety that comes with being invited to show up authentically and ask for what you need, knowing that the professional or organisation is beholden to the core values of acceptance, diversity, equity, and inclusion.

On yet another level, The Safe House may be viewed as a framework for reform, with relevance within education, health, allied health, legal, and government systems. The systemic and practical barriers faced by neurodivergent people are complex. Meaningful change from grass roots to public policy level requires collaboration and integration across multiple disciplines. We need continued critical review of current evidence-based practices with input from the neurodivergent community, wide-spread education (and re-education), and a steadfast commitment to continuous refinement of person-centred models of care. The Safe House is a framework for organising one's thinking around how best to effect change with the aim of creating a society that embraces neurodivergent minds, and values the contributions of people who think and see things differently. It is a mammoth task, and I am by no means claiming to have all the answers. However I would like to participate in the conversation, and offer the Safe House as my small contribution to the cultural shift that is already underway.

3. FOUNDATIONS

The foundation refers to the theory, research, and values which underpin the neurodiversity affirming approach to care. As the neurodiversity paradigm is not (yet) the dominant paradigm, we cannot assume people understand what is meant by the term 'neurodiversity affirming'. The approach differs from traditional approaches to evidence-based practice in relatively small but highly significant ways, and is a paradigm shift for those whose training was couched in the medical model. As such, laying the foundation means providing key stakeholders (parents, carers, teachers, employers, health professionals, therapists, support workers) with education regarding the core values that underpin the neurodiversity affirming approach, and the key concepts and research that support it.

Important Definitions

Neurodiversity (noun): refers to the natural neuro-cognitive variability within the human population, acknowledging the fact that every human has a unique nervous system with a unique combination of abilities and needs.

Neurodiverse (adjective): Neurodiverse is an inclusive term used to describe a group of people with different neurotypes. A group of people with the same neurotype is not neurodiverse

Neurodivergence (noun): Cognitive functioning which is not considered 'typical'. Types of neurodivergence include autism, ADHD, dyslexia, dyscalculia, dysgraphia, dyspraxia, hyperlexia, giftedness, Tourette's syndrome, obsessive compulsive disorder, anxiety, traumatic brain injury, and more.

Neurodivergent (adjective): Describes people who have a neurodivergence. Neurodivergent brains differ from the dominant cultural 'norm'. A person can have multiple forms of neurodivergence, in which case they would be multiply divergent.

Neurotypical (adjective): Describes people with neurological development or functioning that is consistent with societal standards and expectations. Neurotypical brains align with the dominant cultural 'norm'. Also referred to as neuronormative, or the neuromajority.

Autistic (adjective): Describes someone who fulfils diagnostic criteria for autism.

Allistic (adjective): Describes someone who is not autistic, but may experience other forms of neurodivergence.

The Social Model of Disability

The social model of disability emerged in the 1970s as a response to the medical model of disability, which saw disability as an individual problem that needed to be fixed through medical intervention (Hogan, 2019). The focus of the medical approach to care is the provision of treatment aimed at improving functioning of the individual, often without addressing the systemic limitations impacting the individual (Chown, 2017). In contrast, the social model views disability as a socially constructed experience that results from the interaction between an individual with an impairment and a society that is not designed to be inclusive or accommodating of their needs (Oliver, 2013). Barriers to full and meaningful participation may be institutional (i.e., organisational or systemic), environmental (i.e., architectural or physical), attitudinal (i.e., derogatory attitudes or lack of understanding), or communicative (i.e., lack of accommodations for people with communication difficulties). A social model perspective both acknowledges the reality of impairment and its impact on the individual, and challenges society to change in order to accommodate people living with impairment through simple inclusive practices such as universal design (Banes, 2021).

The Neurodiversity Movement

The Neurodiversity movement emerged in the late 1990s and early 2000s, with the rise of the internet providing a platform for neurodivergent folk to connect and share their experiences. The neurodiversity movement is a social justice and civil rights movement, and intersects with the wider disability rights movement, advocating for differences in neurotype to be accepted and respected as a natural variation of the human experience (Singer, 2017). Members of the neurodiversity movement argue that the medical model, which views neurodivergent people as disordered, is harmful and stigmatising. The movement challenges the dominant medical and societal view, and argues that diversity in the way people think, learn, and experience the world is a valuable asset to society (Chapman, 2021). The movement advocates for accessibility and inclusion of neurodivergent folk across all areas of society, such as education, employment, and healthcare. This includes the provision of accommodations and support services that are tailored to the unique needs of neurodivergent people (Runswick-Cole, 2014). The movement actively challenges negative stereotypes and stigmatisation, and promotes a more positive and accurate understanding of neurodiversity. The movement encourages self-advocacy and representation of neurodivergent people, and also fights for support and resources for the families and caregivers, who often play a crucial role in promoting their well-being and inclusion. Lastly, the movement promotes neurodiversity as a source of innovation and creativity, and encourages the use of neurodivergent peoples' talents and abilities in the workplace and society.

Critiques of The Neurodiversity Movement

Any endeavour that challenges the status quo inevitably receives some criticism, and the neurodiversity movement is no different. My sole aim is to provide a framework for implementing neurodiversity affirming care, so I will mention only those criticisms which I consider most relevant to the Safe House Framework. For those interested in exploring the topic I invite you to read the work of Ginny Russell, who authored a Chapter titled 'Critiques of the Neurodiversity Movement' in the book 'Autistic Community and the Neurodiversity Movement: Stories from the Frontline' (Kapp, 2019).

The first criticism relates to language. The terms 'neurotypical' and 'neurodivergent' imply there are two distinct groups. This terminology has the potential to be divisive, fueling identity politics and diverting attention away from more fundamental issues of oppression (Runswick-Cole, 2014). Moreover, the binary is not supported by research. For example, research indicates that ADHD traits are evident throughout the human population, varying in degree from clinically significant to subclinical (Larsson, 2012), as are autistic traits (Steer, 2010). I use the terms neurotypical and neurodivergent for clarity, however I acknowledge the issues herein, and implore readers to remain mindful of the implications of language that dichotomises allied groups. The second criticism of the neurodiversity movement is that it is unrepresentative of all neurodivergent people, and specifically fails to represent autistic folk with high support needs (Russell, 2020). For those who may share this criticism, please be assured that the Safe House Framework has been designed for use with people of all abilities.

4. FLOORPLAN

The floorplan refers to the individual profile of strengths, differences, needs, and abilities of the neurodivergent person. Each human, regardless of neurotype, has a profile of traits and abilities that is as individual and unique as their fingerprint. An understanding of a neurodivergent person's profile is central to the development of their Safe House. A thorough and nuanced profile typically requires input from multiple informants, including the neurodivergent person, people who know them well, and skilled assessment by one or more members of the person's professional team.

Before exploring the subtle nuances within the autistic profile it is worth reviewing the core features of autism. Below is a description of autism as defined by the dominant diagnostic manual, with pathologising language replaced with affirming alternatives. This is followed by an explanation of several common autistic behaviours as serving a self-regulatory function. Lastly, some common stereotypes and myths are addressed.

A word on the problems with diagnoses

The core function of a diagnosis to identify the cause of a particular presentation, and to inform the most appropriate course of action thereafter. Some diagnostic criteria are narrow and highly specific, and point towards a clear protocol for what follows, however this is not the case with autism. The diagnostic criteria for autism are inherently imprecise, and accurate diagnosis requires clinicians with robust knowledge of the criteria, as well as a granular, nuanced understanding of the various ways in which autism presents. For clinicians without autism-specific training it can be challenging to differentiate autism from other diagnoses, and unfortunately misdiagnosis is a common experience for many autistic folk, especially those with atypical or internalised presentations. In fact, limited availability of suitably trained clinicians is one of the most common barriers to diagnosis, along with cost, geographic constraints, and waitlists. And while an autism diagnosis may help with access to funding and supports, it does not necessarily indicate which supports are needed, or what will be most helpful.

What autism *is*

Autism is a neurodevelopmental difference (Monteiro, 2018), with differences appearing in three key areas:

Language and communication

This includes differences in:

- The process of language acquisition and development of speech.
- How speech and language is used.
- The way verbally presented information is processed.
- How non-verbal communication is used and understood.

Social Relationships and Emotional Responses

This includes differences in:

- Social interaction style.
- Awareness of social context and cues.
- Understanding of interpersonal dynamics.
- Emotional awareness (in self and others).
- Capacity for emotional regulation.

Sensory Needs and Interests

This includes:

- Preference for routine.
- Sensory-based movements or behaviours (stims).
- Differences in sensory profile (i.e., hyper- and hypo- sensitivities).
- Areas of passionate interest(s).

Support Needs

An autism diagnosis includes an estimate of the amount of support the diagnosed person requires, expressed as a *level*. People assigned a level one are deemed to *require support*, while those assigned level two *require substantial support*, and those assigned level three *require very substantial support*. The decision around which level to assign is based upon the information obtained throughout the assessment process and is, at best, a rough approximation. The reality of autism is such that support needs are dynamic, varying from day to day, situation to situation, and across the lifespan. Levels are often used to determine a person's access to funding and formal supports, and while still overly simplistic, are most useful in that context.

Preference for Routine

Most people, regardless of neurotype, feel calmer when they know and understand what is coming up next. Many autistic folk have a strong preference for routine and predictability, and this is mostly related to its self-regulatory function. Having a consistent schedule helps to create a predictable and calming environment, which in turn helps to regulate the body's internal rhythms. Routine can also help to manage sensory processing differences by improving the person's ability to cope with sensory input. Moreover, knowing what to expect in most areas of life can help to offset the stress that often accompanies the unpredictability and uncertainty of social interactions.

Stims: Self-Stimulatory Behaviour

Stims are body movements that meet a sensory need and/ or help the person self-regulate. Behaviours like rocking, twirling, flapping, toe walking, and finger flicking are examples of classic stims, but stimming can be any movement or behaviour that a person engages in repeatedly with the aim of meeting a sensory or self-regulatory need, including repeating words or vocalisations, tensing muscles, squeezing, pulling hair, watching a fan spin, smelling objects, lining up items, etc. Stimming is not unique to autism - the behaviour is observed across the population - however it is more frequently observed in autistic folk. Stimming is a common part of the autistic experience, and can serve as a coping mechanism, a form of communication, or a way to regulate sensory input.

Spins: Special Interests, or Passions

These are topics of high interest, and spending time engaged in activities related to these interests is intrinsically rewarding and regulating for the neurodivergent individual. Topics of special interests are often quite specific (i.e., narrow), and are frequently accompanied by great depth of knowledge. A person may have many different special interests, and they may change over time, sometimes very rapidly. Spending time engaged in special interests has a positive effect on well-being, and is frequently the driving force for connections with others who share the same interests. Focusing on SPINS in conversation, sometimes experienced by conversation partners as 'info-dumping', often serves to create a predictable structure in an otherwise unpredictable social exchange.

Monotropism

A monotropic mind is one that focuses its attention on a small number of interests at any one time, and tends not to notice things outside of this attention tunnel. Sometimes referred to as hyper-focus, monotropism lends itself to deep thinking, intense experiences, and flow states (Milton D., 2019). Monotropism is thought to be an adaptive cognitive strategy employed by neurodivergent minds as a means of managing limited availability of attention (Murray, 2005), sensitivity to external stimuli, and difficulty processing multiple sources of information. Monotropism is also posited to be the reason autistic folk tend to be either very interested in something, or not interested at all (Milton D., 2019); where neurotypical minds are more likely to respond to competing attentional demands by splitting their attention (polytropism), neurodivergent minds are more likely to focus intensely on the demand of highest interest and disregard the rest. In fact, the theory of monotropism may be used to explain many common autistic traits, either directly or indirectly. Social interactions, for instance, inherently involve simultaneously processing multiple sources of information, such as speech, gestures, tone, and environmental and sensory demands, while also considering the social norms and expectations, and monitoring one's own response. When viewed through the lens of monotropism, it is unsurprising that neurodivergent folk miss cues and/or are left feeling overwhelmed and tired by social situations. It also explains why social interactions between neurodivergent folk, which tend to be centred around a shared interest or activity, do not encounter the same challenges. Similarly, it makes sense that a hyper-focused mind would need time to adjust to prepare for transitions and adjust to change.

What autism *is not*

Research has driven huge advances in our understanding of neurodiversity over the last 10 -15 years, and some brilliant minds are working tirelessly towards the goal of widespread awareness, acceptance, and inclusion of neurodiverse folk. Despite this progress, myths and stereotypes around neurodiversity in general, and autism in particular, are commonplace. Below are some of the most common areas of misunderstanding:

Myth 1. Autistic people are not interested in relationships.

In truth, many neurodivergent folk are very socially motivated, and given the right supports have deep and fulfilling friendships and relationships. However, the harsh reality is that neurodivergent folk also often come up against more barriers to forming and maintaining relationships. Obvious barriers include rejection by neurotypical peers, communication differences, sensory differences, and a high need for predictability, which can make unstructured social interactions difficult.

Myth 2. Autistic people lack social skills.

The DSM-5-TR (APA, 2013), one of the two most widely accepted classifiers of mental disorders, defines autism as 'a disorder of social communication and behaviour'. Implicit in this definition is the belief that autistic people are responsible for breakdowns in social interactions and communication, with the failure specifically attributed to deficits in social-emotional reciprocity, non-verbal communication skills, empathy, and social skills. However, research has demonstrated that the problem is mutual - the breakdown occurs not only because autistic people have trouble understanding allistic people, but also because allistic people have trouble understanding them. This broadly referred to as the Double Empathy Problem (Milton, 2012), which states that the communication difficulties arise from qualitative differences in the way neurodivergent and neurotypical people communicate, rather than an inherent deficit in the autistic communication partner's ability.

Myth 3. Autistic people lack empathy.

It is true that some neurodivergent folk find it difficult to understand and identify emotions in themselves and others. This is a condition called alexithymia, which affects approximately 10 percent of the general population and approximately 50 percent of autistic people. However, the level of empathy experienced by autistic folk without alexithymia is no different to that of neurotypical folk (Brewer, 2016). Therefore, when people assume that all autistic people lack empathy, they will be wrong 50 percent of the time. For many neurodivergent folk it is differences in the way they experience and respond to empathy which lead others to perceive them as lacking empathy. Moreover, research has demonstrated that some autistic folk have heightened levels of cognitive empathy, which allows for a nuanced and detailed understanding of other's thoughts and feelings (Baron-Cohen, 2001).

Myth 4. Autistic behaviours are weird.

Many of the common autistic behaviours considered to be 'weird', such as stimming and echolalia[2], are human behaviours evident across the population, but which may occur more frequently, and perhaps more overtly, in neurodivergent folk. Labelling them 'autistic behaviours' pathologises normal, harmless behaviours, in effect 'othering' neurodivergent folk and thus increasing the risk of mistreatment. For those interested in exploring this topic in more detail, I recommend the book *Uniquely Human: A Different Way of Seeing Autism* by Barry Prizant.

---

[2]   Echolalia is the immediate or delayed repetition of speech often seen in children learning to talk. In language, a gestalt is a 'chunk' of several words that a speaker hears, memorises, and uses as a whole. Gestalt Language Processing (GLP) is a form of language development that starts with gestalts. GLP is a normal part of language development; all children have some gestalts, even if they mostly start speaking word-by-word. Most autistic children are gestalt language processors. Where allistic children quickly move on to using single words to communicate, autistic children continue tend to continue to use gestalts (i.e., immediate and delayed echolalia).

What goes into constructing a safe house?

Development of an individual profile for an autistic individual begins with understanding their unique presentation of the autistic traits described above. Autism being a spectrum, the variation within the autistic population is immense, giving meaning to the saying 'if you know one autistic person, you know one autistic person'. Beyond the features identified in the diagnostic criteria there are a number of areas in which neurodivergent people commonly experience differences and difficulties. Accurate and timely identification of all areas of need is essential to holistic care and support planning. Below is a list of features to consider:

Sleep

Sleep disturbances and alterations in circadian rhythms are common among autistic folk, and difficulties are genetically and biologically based (Carmassi, 2019). A review of studies investigating the prevalence of sleep problems in autism found that sleep problems are twice as common among neurodivergent children as they are among neurotypical children or those with other developmental differences (Cohen, 2014), with as many as 80 percent of autistic preschoolers experiencing sleep difficulties. Overall autistic folk take longer to fall asleep and wake up more frequently during the night. Sleep is less restorative, with neurodivergent folk spending less of their sleeping time in the rapid eye movement (REM) stage, which is critical for learning and retaining memories (Mannion, 2014). The reasons for poor sleep are varied. Many folk have co-occurring difficulties that contribute to sleep disturbance, such as:

- ADHD, which disrupts sleep in itself, and the stimulant medication for ADHD often causes delayed sleep onset.
- Anxiety, which comes with physiological arousal, worry, and rumination.
- Gastrointestinal problems, which can cause discomfort and pain.
- Sensory sensitivities to light, sound, or touch.
- Sleep problems may be related to depression, though whether depression is the cause or result of sleep difficulties tends to be difficult to determine.
- Sleep apnoea, which affects breathing and causes frequent waking during the night.

Genetic studies have shown that autistic folk are more likely to have mutations in genes that govern the sleep-wake cycle, or those that have links to insomnia (Veatch, 2015). Certainly, one of those mutations is thought to affect levels of melatonin, the natural hormone that controls sleep (Rossignol, 2011). Quality sleep is a basic human need, and sadly one that is often not adequately met for neurodivergent people, often with wide ranging negative effects on daily life. For folk who regularly experience sleep difficulties, identifying and facilitating access to a safe, viable solution needs to be a priority. Given the complexity of sleep problems, consultation with both a psychologist and medical practitioner is recommended.

Questions to ask: What is the quality of sleep for the neurodivergent person? Do they fall asleep and stay asleep without difficulty? Do they sleep soundly? Do they wake feeling refreshed? Are their natural sleep patterns compatible with their lifestyle?

Nutrition

Feeding and eating difficulties (i.e., fear of trying new foods, insistence on specific food presentation, disordered eating) are common among autistic children (Baraskewich, 2021), and to a lesser but still significant extent, adults. A meta-analysis found that autistic children are five times as likely as their neurotypical peers to have an eating concern (Koomar, 2021). For some people, the restricted range of foods eaten limits their ability to meet their nutritional needs through food alone. In extreme cases this poses a significant health risk.

Avoidant and Restrictive Food Intake Disorder (ARFID) is an eating disorder where food intake is restricted, however unlike eating disorders such as anorexia or bulimia, ARFID does not involve a preoccupation with body image or weight. Rather, aversions to food are thought to be related to one or more of the following factors:

- Sensory sensitivities, in particular preference for certain textures, and an aversion to unfamiliar or non-preferred textures and flavours
- Fear of aversive consequences when eating, such as gagging or choking

- A lack of interest in food or eating, which is often related to poor interoception, or limited awareness of the cues for hunger from one's body

ARFID is seen across the lifespan, but it is most commonly diagnosed in children and adolescents, and can have serious consequences if left undetected and/or untreated. Without supplementation, the lack of variety and/or quantity of food consumed often leads to nutritional deficiencies, affecting growth, development, and physical and mental health.

ARFID is considered a mental health condition, however working with ARFID is often complex and requires a multidisciplinary approach, and in the case of children, involves the whole family. For example, in the ideal scenario for a child with ARFID, the team would include:

- a paediatrician, to monitor nutrition levels through blood tests and assess gastrointestinal functioning, and perhaps refer on to a gastroenterologist if need be.

- a dietitian, to guide parents around how best to ensure their child's nutritional needs are met, whether that is with food or supplements.

- a psychologist, to work with the child and family around the psychological factors that are contributing to the condition.

- a speech pathologist, to assess oral motor functions, such as chewing and swallowing.

- an occupational therapist, to assess where sensory differences may be impacting the child.

As with sleep, adequate nutrition is a basic human need, so identifying problems with the variety and quantity of foods consumed, and accessing appropriate supports must be a priority.

Questions to ask: Is food a source of stress or anxiety for the person and/or those caring for them? Does the person eat some food from all the major food groups (i.e., fruits, vegetables, grains, protein foods, dairy)? Do they consume enough food to meet their daily nutritional and energy needs? Are they adequately hydrated?

Gastrointestinal Disorders

Gastrointestinal issues such as constipation, diarrhea, or abdominal pain, and reflux are common among autistic people, with studies reporting that up to 90 percent of folk experience one or more symptoms (Leader, 2022). A systematic review and meta-analysis revealed that autistic people of all ages are significantly more likely to develop inflammatory bowel disease, ulcerative colitis, or Crohn's disease (Kim, 2022), while a large investigation of children suggested that autistic children were approximately 47 percent more likely to be diagnosed with Crohn's disease and 94 percent more likely to be diagnosed with ulcerative colitis compared with controls (Lee, 2018). Of particular concern is the fact that autistic children often have difficulty articulating and describing symptoms like abdominal pain, however without treatment, symptoms may have a significant impact on their overall health and well-being. For this reason it is important that parents and carers' are aware of their child's general gut health.

The high rate of gastrointestinal issues in autistic populations has generated interest and research into the possible role of the gut-brain connection. The gut-brain connection refers to the communication and feedback loop between the gastrointestinal system and the central nervous system, which includes the brain and spinal cord. The gut has its own complex nervous system, known as the enteric nervous system, consisting of over 100 million neurons that control the function of the digestive tract. The enteric nervous system can function independently of the central nervous system, but it also communicates with the brain via the vagus nerve, a long nerve that connects the brainstem to the abdomen. Through this communication network, the gut and the brain can influence each other's function and activity. For example, when we feel stressed or anxious, our brain sends signals to the gut which can lead to symptoms such as nausea, stomach pain, or diarrhea. Similarly, diet and the gut microbiome can affect our mood, cognition, and behaviour.

The gut microbiome refers to the collection of microorganisms, including bacteria, viruses, fungi, and other microbes, that live in the digestive tract of humans and other animals. The gut microbiome plays a crucial role in maintaining human health by helping to digest food, produce vitamins and fatty acids, and regulate the immune system. A balanced microbial composition is important to health, as dysbiosis - a disruption in the normal diversity and abundance of the microbes that make up the gut microbiome – has been shown to be related to a arrange of conditions, such as inflammatory bowel disease, irritable bowel syndrome, Alzheimer's disease, and type 2 diabetes mellitus.

Research has demonstrated significant changes in microbial composition of autistic populations, in particular decreased bacterial diversity compared to allistic populations, with fewer beneficial bacteria, and more pathogenic bacteria (Srikantha, 2019). More studies are needed to fully understand the relationship between the microbiome and autism, however research investigating various interventions that target gut health (i.e., prebiotic and probiotic supplementation) in autistic people certainly suggests that this is an area worthy of exploration (Taniya, 2022). For those interested, this falls within the scope of a general medical practitioner, integrative or functional medical practitioner, or naturopath.

Questions to ask: Does the person experience gastrointestinal distress (i.e., pain, reflex) regularly? Does the person have healthy bowel functioning (see https://www.continence.org.au/bristol-stool-chart for a guide).

Muscle tone

Low muscle tone, called hypotonia, is more common in autistic infants and children than their neurotypical peers (Ludyga, 2021), leading to gross and fine motor difficulties, poor posture, fatigue, and pain, often with negative impacts on functional capacity and emotional wellbeing. Timely identification and physiotherapy is important to minimise the impact of low tone on physical development.

Questions to ask: For very young children, do they appear 'floppy' when being held? Do they have difficulty feeding or swallowing? Are their gross motor (i.e., rolling, sitting, crawling, walking) and fine motor (i.e., holding, grabbing, pinching) skills developing within the expected timeframes? For children, does the child appear to have poor posture? Do they find it difficult to stand or sit unsupported for long periods of time? Are they overly flexible? Are their reflexes slower than expected for their age? Do they have poor endurance?

Sensory profile

Sensory processing refers to the brain's ability to register, organise, and make sense of information received via the senses. Sensory processing differences are observed in as many as 90 percent of autistic folk (Ben-Sasson, 2009). Increased sensitivity (also called hyper-sensitivity, or high registration) or decreased sensitivity (also called hypo-sensitivity, or low registration) may present in relation to one or more of the following sensory systems:

1. The visual system is responsible for seeing. Sensory processing differences in the visual system include differences in sensitivity to light, colour, pattern, depth, orientation, and movement.

2. The auditory system is responsible for hearing. Sensory processing differences in the auditory system refers to differences in sensitivity to sound.

3. The olfactory system is responsible for processing smell. Sensory processing differences in the olfactory system refers to differences in sensitivity to odour.

4. The gustatory system is responsible for processing taste. Sensory processing differences in the gustatory system refers to differences in sensitivity to flavours.

5. The tactile system is responsible for processing touch information from the body. Sensory processing differences in the tactile system refers to differences in sensitivity to touch and texture.

6. The vestibular system is responsible for informing us about the movement and position of our head in space. Sensory processing differences in the vestibular system refers to differences in sensitivity to movement and equilibrium (i.e., balance).

7. The proprioceptive system is responsible for informing us about the position, location, orientation, and movement of one's body parts. Sensory processing differences proprioception refers to differences in perception or awareness of the position and movement of one's body.

8. The interoceptive system is responsible for informing us about the physiological responses that guide regulation, such as hunger, thirst, pain, and temperature. Interoception is also involved in emotional awareness and regulation. Sensory processing differences in interoception refers to differences in sensitivity to internal bodily cues.

Sensory processing differences are highly individual and may fluctuate between situations and over time. A thorough assessment of a person's sensory profile by an occupational therapist is often useful when looking to identify the most appropriate supports for sensory processing differences.

Questions to ask: Is the person highly sensitive to one or more aspects of their environment, such as light, noise, or odour? Does the person avoid certain sensory experiences, such as specific food textures, or physical affection? Do they seek out certain sensory experiences to self-regulate, such as deep pressure, or vigorous movement? Do they appear clumsy or uncoordinated? Do they notice cues from their body that they are hungry, thirsty, or cold? In children, do they have toileting accidents that seem to stem from a lack of bodily awareness?

Executive Functions

Executive functioning skills refers to the brain-based skills responsible for regulating goal-directed, future-oriented tasks, and include mental behaviours such as planning, organising, maintaining attention, prioritising, and regulating emotions and behaviour. Executive functions are akin to an orchestra conductor, whose role it is to choose the music, decide how it will be played, set the tempo for the orchestra, and direct each section of the orchestra to play at the right time (Brown, 2006). In the same way, executive functions allow us to self-regulate by cueing, directing, and coordinating the various mental skills needed in everyday activities. In short, executive functions are responsible for the mental management of finite resources. They are the part of our brain function that helps us *get stuff done*.

Executive functions can be broken down into three core processes (Miyake, 2000):

1. Working memory: refers to the ability to retain and manipulate information over short periods of time.
2. Set shifting or cognitive flexibility: refers to the ability to maintain or shift focus and attention in response to different demands, rules, or settings.
3. Response inhibition or self control: refers to the ability to resist impulsive actions and set priorities.

Executive functioning difficulties are common in neurodivergent folk (Lai, 2017), and can interfere with self-care, independence, learning, employment, and relationships. The unfortunate reality for many people is that a lack of understanding of executive functions results in them being labelled lazy and or unmotivated. With such pervasive impacts, executive functioning difficulties are often a source of significant stress and anxiety. When individual differences in executive functions are accurately identified, supports can be put in place to mitigate or minimise the impact on the individual's activities of daily living.

Questions to ask: Does the person seem inattentive, spacey, forgetful, or distractible? Does the person have trouble organising their belongings? Do they find it difficult to set goals and work towards them? Do they have difficulty estimating how long a task will take? Do they find it hard to get started on tasks? Do they tend to act impulsively? Do they experience intense emotions? Do they find it difficult to regulate their emotions and behaviour? Do they tend to hyper-focus on activities that are of high interest, yet find themselves unable to focus on low-interest tasks?

Communication

Differences in speech and language development, ability, and style are a core feature of autism, and understanding the extent to which an autistic person is able to effectively use language to communicate is essential to ensuring their interactions with others are experienced as safe. This is especially relevant when working with children, whose speech and language development may be delayed or atypical.

Language can be broken down into three key areas:

- Receptive Language: the ability to understand language that is spoken, written, or signed by others. It involves the processing of sounds, words, sentences, and other forms of communication in order to derive meaning.

- Expressive Language: the ability to communicate thoughts, ideas, and emotions through spoken, written, or signed language. It involves using words, sentences, and other forms of communication to convey a message.

- Pragmatic Language: the social use of language in communication, including the ability to use language appropriately in different social contexts, to understand and follow conversational rules, and to interpret nonverbal cues.

VALLI JONES

It is common for a person's ability to vary between areas of language, and many autistic folk find that their ability to communicate using language is affected by their emotional state. Assessment by a speech and language pathologist is recommended in order to fully understand an individual's communication ability.

Questions to ask: What is the person's ability to understand language (receptive language skills)? What is the person's ability to use language to communicate (expressive language skills)? What is the person's ability to adjust their language to suit different social situations (pragmatic language skills)? Does the person's ability to use and/or understand language reduce when they are stressed or upset? Are they very literal in their interpretation of language? Do they recognise when someone is using sarcasm? Do they appear to detect changes in someone's tone of voice? To what extent does the person effectively use non-verbal communication (i.e., facial expression and body language)? To what extent does the person pick up on non-verbal communication from others?

Minimally verbal and non-speaking folk

For people with limited ability to effectively communicate their needs, wishes, and experiences, timely access to intervention and supports is a basic need and fundamental human right. For minimally verbal and non-speaking autistics, the following questions are relevant:

Questions to ask: Does the person have access to assistive technology to communicate (i.e., communication boards, electronic devices)? Are they able to use the assistive technology effectively? Is the assistive technology the option that is best suited to their needs, ability, and context? Is their ability to communicate effectively limited by the specific technology? Are all important members of the person's support team trained to use the assistive technology effectively? For people who use multiple modes of communication, what is their preferred mode?

Cognition

Cognitive ability, sometimes referred to as intelligence, broadly refers to one's ability to think, reason, and learn. An assessment of cognitive ability can be a useful tool when there are concerns around a person's ability to process information, understand concepts, and/or apply knowledge appropriately. Cognitive test results provide information about overall ability, and also break overall ability down into sub-categories of ability.

To illustrate, one of the commonly used instruments for children measures the following cognitive abilities (note: similar assessment tools are available for use with adults, and produce comparable information):

• Overall ability (Full Scale Intelligence Quotient, or FSIQ). This is considered a broad representation of a child's cognitive ability. The FSIQ score is the combined result of scores from tests of five areas of cognitive ability, described below. Some children perform at approximately the same level in all areas, but most neurodivergent children have what is called a 'spiky profile', meaning that their ability varies significantly between areas of cognitive ability. Identifying areas of strength and difficulty can be helpful when seeking to understand how best to support a child in all areas of life, and particularly in relation to schooling.

- Verbal Comprehension. This is a measure of a child's ability to access and apply acquired word knowledge. Specifically, this score reflects a child's ability to verbalise meaningful concepts, think about verbal information, and express oneself using words.

- Visual Spatial Ability. This is measure of a child's ability to evaluate visual details and understand visual spatial relationships in order to construct geometric designs from a model. This skill requires visual spatial reasoning, integration and synthesis of part-whole relationships, attentiveness to visual detail, and visual-motor integration.

- Fluid Reasoning. This is a measure of a child's ability to detect the underlying conceptual relationship among visual objects and use reasoning to identify and apply rules. Identification and application of conceptual relationships requires inductive and quantitative reasoning, broad visual intelligence, simultaneous processing, and abstract thinking.

- Working Memory. This is a measure of a child's ability to register, maintain, and manipulate visual and auditory information in conscious awareness. This requires attention and concentration, as well as visual and auditory discrimination.

- Processing Speed. This is a measure of a child's speed and accuracy of visual identification, decision making, and decision implementation. Performance is related to visual scanning, visual discrimination, short-term visual memory, visuomotor coordination, attention, and concentration. These subtests assess a child's ability to rapidly identify, register, and implement decisions about visual stimuli.

Areas of strength and limitation (i.e., a spiky profile) are especially common among neurodivergent children. In particular, a cognitive assessment often reveals relative limitations in working memory and processing speed. Fortunately, there are specific adjustments and accommodations that educators can put in place to minimise the impact of these cognitive differences on learning. When applied consistently, supports can help a child cope with what might otherwise feel like an unmanageable, overwhelming experience.

It is important to note that while cognitive test scores are often helpful when trying to understand how to support a person's learning, they do not take into account abilities such as emotional intelligence, kinaesthetic awareness, social awareness, moral development, or motivation. When given too much importance, 'intelligence' as a concept may be misleading and obstructive. However, when used appropriately, and within the context of a holistic evaluation, cognitive testing does provide data that may be helpful in informing supports. Cognitive assessment falls within the scope of a psychologist.

Thinking Styles

Thinking styles refer to the specific ways in which an individual approaches problem-solving and decision-making. Some common examples of thinking styles include:

- Convergent thinking, which involves narrowing down multiple options to find a single, correct solution.
- Divergent thinking, which involves generating multiple ideas and possibilities.
- Lateral thinking, which involves approaching a problem or situation in an unconventional way.
- Analytical thinking, which involves breaking down a problem into smaller parts and examining each part in detail.
- Creative thinking, which involves generating new and unique ideas.

Neurodivergent folk tend to process information differently, and there are some thinking styles or characteristics that are more common among neurodivergent folk:

- Literal thinking: a tendency to think in a very concrete and literal way. Literal thinkers may have difficulty understanding idioms, metaphors, jokes, sarcasm, and other forms of figurative language.

- Black-and-white thinking: a tendency to see things in terms of right and wrong, or good and bad. Black and white thinkers may have difficulty seeing nuances or exceptions, and this can make it difficult to understand complex issues and make decisions.

- Rigid thinking: a tendency toward inflexible thinking, rigid thinkers have a hard time adapting to changes or new ideas, and considering alternatives or different perspectives.

- Holistic thinking: a tendency to see the big picture and think in an integrated manner. Holistic thinkers may have difficulty focusing on details, or breaking things down into smaller parts. Holistic thinking makes it difficult to follow detailed instructions, or complete tasks that require step-by-step thinking.

- Hyper-focus: a tendency to become absorbed in a specific task or interest. Hyper-focused thinkers may lose track of time and have difficulty switching to other tasks. Hyper-focus can be beneficial when completing projects or tasks that require deep concentration but can also lead to difficulties in multitasking or completing other responsibilities.

- Divergent thinking: divergent thinkers can generate many ideas, and tend to think in a creative, non-linear manner. Divergent thinking can be beneficial in problem-solving and innovation, but it can also make it difficult for people to stay focused on a task and make decisions.

It is important to note that these thinking styles are not exclusive to neurodivergent minds, however many autistic folk have quite distinct patterns in their thought processes, and it can be helpful to identify these. Thinking styles are not inherently positive or negative, rather they are a reflection of how an individual's brain processes information.

Emotion-Regulation and Co-Regulation

As a psychologist working with neurodivergent children, I can count on one hand the number of times emotion-regulation has *not* been listed as an area of concern by a parent or teacher. Emotion-regulation involves the use of various strategies and skills to manage one's internal state and behaviour, and these are underpinned by executive functions. As the act of emotion-regulation is dependent on executive functions, and develops with maturity, it is reasonable to expect all children to need help with emotion-regulation. Autistic children often need more help, and for longer, than their neurotypical peers, and many autistic adults continue to benefit from support.

Research has consistently shown that children learn to self-regulate through repeated co-regulation with a caregiver who is sensitive to the emotional experience of the child. When an attuned adult is able to meet a child's big emotions with a kind and reassuring presence, the adult's mature nervous system will help the child's developing nervous system to regulate. Through repeated experiences of having one's emotions named and validated, and having a caring adult act as an anchor while being tossed around by waves of intense feeling, children gradually learn how to manage their emotions independently.

How best to co-regulate with a child depends on the nature of the relationship between the adult and child (i.e., parent, teacher, therapist), and the characteristics of both the child and the adult. Co-regulation is both a mindset and a skill, and while some adults find it comes naturally, there are an equal number of adults who find themselves feeling lost, powerless, and overwhelmed by a child's big emotions. I see immense value in basic education in the neuroscience and practical application of co-regulation for parents, educators, and other adults charged with caring for children. A key component of such education is self-care, as a dysregulated adult is less able to co-regulate a distressed child. Moreover, the demands of caring for children can be immense, and without adequate regular self-care, are unsustainable.

With the importance of co-regulation in mind, it is worth considering how best to make use of 'chill out zones' and 'calm down corners', often found in homes, classrooms, and inclusive education hubs. There is no doubt value in having a low-stimulation space for children to retreat to when they are feeling overwhelmed. And there may be value in suggesting that some children go to such a space when they are experiencing big emotions. However, many children, when faced with overwhelming emotions, need the human-to-human support of a caring adult who is available to meet them in their distress, and stay with them until it has passed. Without co-regulation many children are simply unable to regulate big emotions, and while they may return to a state that outwardly appears calm, their internal experience is often still turbulent, and the opportunity for learning vital emotion-regulation skills is lost. A better option might be for a caring adult to join the child in the calm zone, where they can offer a calm presence, and an attitude of collaboration and support, whatever that looks like in the moment.

Most children, regardless of neurotype, benefit from the support of co-regulation, however there will be some autistic children who prefer to be alone when upset. As long as solitude is their choice, there is no issue – meet their need for solitude. However, for a child who does not choose solitude, being left alone to cope with overwhelming emotions has the potential to be scary and painful.

Co-occurring Diagnoses

Autism rarely presents in isolation, with the majority of autistic folk having at least one co-occurring condition. According to the scientific literature, as many as 85 percent of autistic people experience a co-occurring anxiety disorder (Postorino, 2017), while 50 percent to 70 percent of people with autism also present with co-occurring attention deficit hyperactivity disorder (Hours, 2022). Other common co-occurrences include obsessive compulsive disorder, learning disorders, depression, intellectual disability, tic disorder, feeding and eating disorders, and epilepsy. A comprehensive evaluation by a suitably trained mental health professional is necessary to accurately identify co-occurring conditions, and to formulate a treatment plan which takes into account other aspects of the individual's profile.

Anxiety

Eighty-five out of every one hundred autistic people experience clinically significant anxiety at some stage of their life. That rate is extremely high. The reasons for such high prevalence are manifold, and individual biological differences certainly play a significant role with research demonstrating reduced flexibility in the nervous systems of neurodivergent people, the result of which is a heightened stress response, and slower recovery after exposure to stress (Fenning, 2019).

My observation has been that the experience of anxiety is often related, directly or indirectly, to a poor fit between person and environment, combined with inadequate accommodations and supports. Sadly, there is a paucity of quality research specifically examining the effectiveness of environmental accommodations in reducing anxiety. Anecdotal reports from the autistic community are certainly consistent with my observation, and preliminary evidence aligns; for example, a 2019 study demonstrated a reduction in sympathetic activation among noise-sensitive autistic children who were provided with noise-attenuating headphones (Pfeiffer, 2019). However, the overwhelming majority of research investigating interventions aimed at reducing anxiety among autistic populations has focused on pharmacological and/or psychological treatment. To ensure the need for environmental accommodations is met, we need more high quality research in this area, and empirical support.

Given the ubiquity of anxiety among autistic people, it is relevant to make specific mention of the various manifestations, which vary between people, and also between contexts within the same person. Some common ways anxiety presents include:

- Increased stimming.
- Avoidance of social situations.
- Demand avoidance, stemming from an increased need for control.
- Physical symptoms such as stomach-aches, headaches, or difficulty sleeping.
- Difficulty communicating; otherwise communicative folk may not be able to speak, or may have difficulty initiating or participating in conversations.
- Heightened sensory sensitivities and/or sensory overwhelm.
- Aggressive or self-injurious behaviour.
- Shutdowns
- Meltdowns

Having people around who recognise the signs of anxiety and support the neurodivergent person to self-regulate is extremely important for many folk, especially children. I believe practical training in this area is essential for all educators and professionals working with neurodiverse groups of children (i.e., all populations of children), to ensure that anxiety related behaviours are not mistakenly attributed to defiance, thereby attracting punitive consequences. Even more so, I advocate for provisions of individual accommodations and support, which I observe to significantly reduce the anxiety experienced by many autistic children. Workplaces with neurodivergent staff members would similarly benefit from routine training in this area.

The Neurodivergent Nervous System

Research suggests that the neurodivergent nervous system functions differently, with higher rates of autonomic dysregulation (i.e., stress) observed in neurodivergent folk (Arora, 2021). To explain this, some context is required. The nervous system involves two different systems; the central nervous system (CNS), which includes the brain and spinal cord, and the peripheral nervous system (PNS), which carries information between the body and the CNS. The PNS is what connects the body and brain, and so is central to the body-brain connection. The PNS consists of two branches; the somatic nervous system (SNS), which voluntarily controls movement, and the autonomic nervous system (ANS), which controls internal processes such as heart and breathing rate, blood pressure, body temperature, digestion, metabolism, and sexual arousal. Within the ANS there are two subsystems; the sympathetic nervous system and the parasympathetic nervous system. In terms of understanding the differences in the neurodivergent nervous system, the sympathetic and parasympathetic systems are of particular interest.

The sympathetic and parasympathetic systems control the same organs, however, they have opposing roles. The sympathetic mode is the accelerator (i.e., fight or flight mode) and the parasympathetic mode is the brake (i.e., rest and digest mode). Through a process called neuroception, the ANS assesses the environment for potential danger and responds accordingly, often before conscious awareness. When functioning optimally, the sympathetic and parasympathetic systems work in harmony to activate the 'fight or flight' mode when danger is detected, and restore calm in the absence of danger. A healthy nervous system is flexible, and able to adapt to shifts in the internal or external environment in order to maintain equilibrium.

In neurodivergent people, the 'fight or flight' branch of the ANS tends to be more easily activated (i.e., is more sensitive to stressors, and detects cues for danger more readily) and takes longer to return to a state of equilibrium (i.e., is more rigid). In practical terms, this equates to a more frequent and heightened stress response, with more cortisol and adrenalin circulating in the body over longer periods of time. Given that neurodivergent folk tend to encounter stressors more frequently, such as difficulties arising due to differences in communication style, executive functioning, and sensory profile, or any number of systemic barriers, the reality is that many neurodivergent people spend a great deal of their time in a stressed, sympathetic state. This has negative short- and long- term impacts on mental and physical health, increases vulnerability to trauma, and underlies what is commonly referred to as autistic burnout.

With self-awareness and a comprehensive self-care regime, many neurodivergent people are able to minimise the impact of their sensitive and rigid nervous system. Often this involve ensuring that the necessary supports and accommodations are consistently in place, reducing demands, implementing regular practices such as breathwork to improve vagal tone (i.e., increase the flexibility of the ANS), and creating a lifestyle that supports regular deep rest. The unfortunate reality is that most neurodivergent people do not have the support or time necessary for such a self-care plan, and so find themselves in a 'boom-bust' cycle of chronic sympathetic nervous system overactivation, followed by burnout.

Demand Avoidance (Anxiety-Driven Need for Control)

Pathological Demand Avoidance, or Pervasive Drive for Autonomy (PDA) is common among neurodivergent folk. Also referred to as 'Pervasive' or 'Extreme' Demand Avoidance, this is often considered a distinct profile of autism characterised by extreme resistance to external, and at times internal, demands (O'Nions, 2018). Demand avoidant behaviour is underpinned by anxiety, whereby demands activate the sympathetic nervous system, manifesting as an intense need for control (Stuart, 2020). Examples of demands include:

- Directions, instruction, questions, and requests from others.
- Explicit expectations from self and others (e.g., deadlines).

- Implied expectations (e.g., praise, which implies that the behaviour needs to be repeated).

- The need to make a decision.

- Uncertainty, which comes with a perceived lack of control.

- Internal bodily demands (e.g., hunger, thirst, fatigue).

- Transitions.

- Sensory overwhelm.

- The wants and needs of others.

- One's own wants and needs.

- Self-care tasks (e.g., showering, teeth brushing, toileting)

Demands are perceived differently by different people, and demand avoidance occurs on a spectrum, tending to increase during times of stress. Demand avoidance may present as withdrawal, refusal, shutdown, or meltdown, though often more socially astute responses such as distraction, procrastination, or excuses are attempted first, followed by more extreme measures such as withdrawing into fantasy, or aggression towards self or others (O'Nions, 2016).

While there has been a great deal of controversy surrounding the validity of PDA as a classifier or diagnostic term, the practical utility in understanding how and why demand avoidant behaviour presents is undeniable for those experiencing it, as well as those living and/or working with demand avoidant folk (Ozsivadjian, 2020). Similarly, understanding what is required to both minimise anxiety, and accommodate the autistic person's need for control, as well as how best to respond to demand avoidant behaviour, is crucial in creating a sense of safety. My observation has been that appropriate accommodation of individual differences (e.g., communication, sensory, cognitive) along with pre-emptive opportunities for choice and control are helpful in reducing the frequency and intensity of demand avoidance, while compassion, humour, and flexibility tend to be the most helpful responses when demand avoidant behaviour occurs. The United Kingdom based PDA Society is a helpful starting point for those seeking more information. https://www.pdasociety.org.uk

Twice Exceptionality

'Twice exceptional', or 2e, is a term used to describe people who have both exceptional abilities *and* disabilities. Twice exceptional or multiply exceptional people have both areas of exceptional strength (i.e., intelligence or creativity) as well as areas of difficulty (i.e., autism, ADHD, or learning difficulties). For example, a person may be considered twice exceptional if they have a high IQ and are gifted in a certain area, such as math or music, but are also autistic and experience the difficulties therein. Twice exceptionality can be particularly challenging to accurately identify and support, as the exceptional abilities of 2e folk may mask their areas of difficulty, and conversely, their areas of difficulty may mask their exceptional abilities. Many 2e folk are not adequately supported in traditional gifted programs, nor in inclusive education programs. Consequently, 2e people are too often overlooked and under-served, and tend to require specialised assessment and support to flourish.

Gender Identity

Numerous studies indicate a relationship exists between gender diversity and autism (Strang, 2018). Compared to cisgender people, transgender and gender-diverse people have, on average, higher rates of autism, other neurodivergences, and psychiatric diagnoses. Irrespective of neurotype, transgender and gender-diverse people tend to score higher on self-report measures of autistic traits, systemizing, and sensory sensitivity, and somewhat lower on self-report measures of empathy (Warrier, 2020). While the precise relationship between gender identity and autism is unclear, the practical implication of these findings is that autistic folk are more likely to identify as gender diverse (i.e., transgender, nonbinary, or gender-queer). This places autistic gender diverse folk at the intersection of two minority groups with all the marginalisation inherent within, without considering any of the many other challenges the individual may face. We know that gender diverse folk and autistic folk are independently more likely to experience depression, anxiety, and suicidality (Biggs, 2022) and the combined effect of belonging to both groups is compounded. One of the most important factors influencing mental health outcomes is the degree of affirmation and support from family and friends, however the unfortunate reality is that many parents of gender diverse children are unsure of how to respond when their child shares their news, and unintentionally cause harm by responding with concern or dismissiveness. At the most basic level, it is essential neurodiversity affirming care includes an attitude of acceptance and respect with regard to preferred pronouns, preferred name, sexuality, and provides education for family members as needed. The following resource is a good starting point:

https://www.orygen.org.au/Training/Resources/ trans-and-gender-diverse-young-people/Videos/ Journeys-Affirming-gender-diversity-in-young-people

Intellectual Disability

Intellectual disability (ID), also known as cognitive impairment, commonly co-occurs with autism. Prevalence rates vary significantly between studies, with estimates ranging from 29 percent (Rydzewska, 2019) to 55 percent (Charman, 2011) depending on the study. Folk with co-occurring intellectual disability typically require some degree of support across all areas of daily living, though the level of support required depends heavily upon the severity of impairment. Intellectual disability is identified through an assessment of both cognitive and adaptive functioning, which is generally completed by a psychologist.

Strengths

A neurodivergent person's unique strengths and abilities are as relevant to the development of their Safe House as their areas of difficulty, in that they provide an avenue for fostering joy, success, resilience, and wellbeing. Individual strengths are incredibly varied, and are best identified using a combination of self-report, interview, direct observation, and standardised assessment, and perhaps by reviewing records where appropriate (i.e., school reports). Strengths may include broad or specific cognitive abilities, creativity, adaptive skills, character traits, knowledge and skills in areas of special interest, and any other domain in which a relative strength exists. The range strengths possessed by autistic people is infinite. Below is a tiny sample of strengths I have observed to be common among autistic folk:

- High attention to detail.
- Ability to focus deeply on specific interests.
- Strong memory and recall abilities.
- Good at pattern recognition and visual problem solving.
- Keen sense of integrity, honesty, and justice.
- Good at understanding systems and logic.
- Good at visualising complex information.
- Strong sense of empathy, especially towards animals and nature.
- Creativity, and an appreciation for art.

Masking

Masking, sometimes referred to as compensation or camouflaging, is the act of concealing aspects of oneself in order to pass as 'normal' in everyday social interaction (Hull, 2017). Masking is a strategy employed by many neurodivergent folk as a means of conforming to social expectations. Examples include making forced eye contact, mirroring, hiding or minimizing personal interests, developing a repertoire of rehearsed responses to questions, pushing through intense sensory discomfort, and disguising stimming behaviours.

When we consider that social discord is broadly attributed to the apparent deficits within the autistic way of being, the strategy makes perfect sense. In fact, traditional therapeutic goals for neurodivergent people are often, in one way or another, to 'appear more neurotypical'. Depending on the culture and context in which the neurodivergent person finds themselves, appearing neurotypical may be necessary for acceptance, and in some cases, survival (Pearson, 2021). However, the effort to hide one's authentic self comes at a significant cost. Masking is related to increased levels of exhaustion, burnout, anxiety, depression, and suicidality (Cage, 2019). Identifying masking behaviours and quantifying the extent to which someone is actively working to fit in with their surrounds is important when constructing their individual profile.

Why do we need a Safe House?

As you can see, the internal experience of autism is multifaceted, and varies enormously between people, and also within the same individual over time, and depending on context. On any given day an individual may be impacted by multiple factors, with a cumulative effect on functioning and wellbeing. To illustrate, imagine a child with the common neurodivergent profile of auditory sensitivities, slower processing speed, and receptive language difficulties.

That child will experience noise as a stressor, require longer than their peers to process information and act on it, and will have a limited understanding of both verbal and written communication.

Now imagine that child in a classroom with one teacher and twenty-five other children. From this perspective, it is easy to see how the cumulative effect of being in a noisy, language-laden environment, where the agenda is for all students to work to the same schedule, has the potential to lead to overwhelm and anxiety. A self-aware child might choose to withdraw from the classroom in an attempt to self-regulate (assuming they are permitted to do so), and while this may be helpful on one level, on another level the missed lesson will further impact their already impacted learning. A child who is still learning to recognise their internal cues for overwhelm and anxiety, or who is not permitted to withdraw, might stay in the classroom until they reach the point of shut down or meltdown, at which time they may behave in ways that are considered inappropriate or unacceptable, and which are met with confusion and/or frustration from peers and adults. In either case, the child's experience is negative.

However, if the same child is supported to use noise-reducing ear plugs or headphones, given fewer tasks and/or more time to complete them, and provided information in simple language with visual aides, their experience of the classroom is likely to be vastly improved. Moreover, when not contending with overwhelm and anxiety the child will be better equipped to participate in class activities and learn.

There are countless examples like the one above which illustrate the power and simplicity of effective support planning. The Safe House is a tool that guides the collection of information about individual differences, difficulties, and needs, with the aim of synthesising the information into a holistic schedule of accommodations and supports. By putting appropriate supports in place, we can address many of the barriers to inclusion encountered by autistic folk.

The Safe House Framework also draws attention to interventions which have an evidence-base, but which are inherently problematic when viewed through a neurodiversity affirming lens. The first of these is Applied Behaviour Analysis (ABA), which is still widely considered the 'gold standard intervention' for autism. For those who are unfamiliar with ABA, the approach uses the behavioural learning principles of operant conditioning to shape behaviour.[3] Children prescribed ABA may be required to participate in intensive treatment regimens of upwards of 30 hours per week of early intervention, inevitably at the expense of critically important unstructured play. Supporters of ABA argue that it increases 'socially important' behaviours and reduces or eliminates 'problem' behaviours in autistic children, and advise parents to engage their newly diagnosed child in ABA therapy as soon as possible to give them the

---

[3]   Operant conditioning is a method of learning in which the consequences of a response determine the probability of it being repeated. Through operant conditioning, behaviour which is followed by pleasant consequences (reinforcement) will likely be repeated, and behaviour which is followed by unpleasant consequences will occur less frequently (Skinner, 1963).

best possible start in life. However, the history of ABA is deeply troubling, with the earliest form of the therapy using electric shock and spanking to eliminate unwanted behaviours (Lovaas, 1973). While the practice of ABA has no doubt changed significantly since its inception, the modality still aims for behavioural compliance and conformity, at times disregarding consent, and systematically withholding items or experiences that are important to the child until they perform the desired behaviour - an experience that inadvertently renders them vulnerable to future coercion (Kaylene, 2022). Many autistic adults, parents of autistic children, and therapists have understandably come to view ABA as a highly questionable intervention, with the most ardent critics arguing that it is a dehumanising, traumatic, and abusive practice. Certainly, the accounts of those with lived experience confirm that long-term ABA caused them serious and life-long harms, fracturing the individual's sense of autonomy and resulting in ongoing impairment due to trauma-induced mental illness (Leaf, 2022). For these reasons, ABA therapy is not considered neurodiversity affirming, and is not welcome in the Safe House.

Beyond ABA, operant principles are routinely used to shape behaviour with less frequency and intensity in many homes, classrooms, and therapy clinics. The practice is not called ABA in those settings however the same concerns apply, though often to a lesser extent. Any time rewards such as sweets, free play, or technology time are used to encourage desirable behaviour, either as an incentive (i.e., planned reward) or a spontaneous response, operant conditioning is being used. Similarly, operant principles are being employed any time those same rewards are withheld or removed as a consequence for a failure to behave in a certain manner (i.e., punishment). My intent is not to demonise the use of behavioural strategies; for decades it was thought to be the right thing to do, and culturally many people are so accustomed to using reward and punishment in child rearing and education that to remove it from the 'toolkit' may initially seem like a daunting proposition. I understand that parents and teachers are charged with what sometimes feels like an impossible feat. As a working solo parent of two there were absolutely times that I incentivised (bribed?) my children to get out of the house on time, and having spent time in early childhood and primary school settings I fully appreciate the role rewards can play in managing the competing demands of a busy classroom. The invitation to readers is to be mindful and intentional when caring for children, and to consider all the options available rather than arbitrarily using reward and punishment as a behaviour management tool. Alternative perspectives on behaviour will be discussed later, in the Windows section of the Safe House Framework.

Social skills training is another evidence-based intervention for autism that is widely used in therapy clinics and schools. The goal of social skills training is to equip the neurodivergent person with the skills necessary to meet neurotypical standards for social interactions. The obvious issue is the implication that it is the sole responsibility of the minority group to adjust to the norms of the majority group. In my opinion, it would be more helpful to provide neurotypical people with education in the communication and social differences that exist within neurodivergence, thereby cultivating understanding and acceptance of *all* ways of being. At an individual level, autistic folk describe the experience of social skills training as a demeaning practice that inhibits authenticity, and leads to anxiety, self-consciousness, self-doubt, self-shaming, and hypervigilance. By setting an expectation for autistic folk to conform to neurotypical ideals, social skills training demands the neurodivergent person expend energy masking their autistic traits, a task that is unrealistic for many, and harmful for all. As such, social skills training is not considered neurodiversity affirming, and like ABA, is not welcome in the Safe House.

The obvious exception is when a neurodivergent person identifies social skill development as a personal goal, in which case the skills being sought tend to be more accurately described as relational intelligence skills. Also, when working with children of any neurotype, some explicit teaching around social and emotional wellbeing is beneficial. The problem with social skills training arises when it is applied arbitrarily, based on the assumption that there is a deficit within the neurodivergent way of being, and requiring neurodivergent folk to conform to neurotypical norms.

5. WALLS

The walls of the Safe House refers to the team of people supporting the neurodivergent individual. For a child or adolescent, the team is usually led by parents, and includes extended family members or adult friends with whom the child has developed a close and trusting relationship, as well as teachers, teacher aides, therapists (e.g., psychologist, speech pathologist, occupational therapist, physiotherapist, dietitian), medical professionals (e.g., general practitioner, paediatrician, psychiatrist), and paid carers. In short, *everyone* who is routinely involved in providing care, services, and supports to the child and their family.

For an adult the team may be different, influenced by factors such as the presence and availability of family members, friendships, intimate relationships, support needs, level of social participation, employment status, and living arrangements. In essence though, the same principle applies; everyone who is routinely involved in providing care, services, and support is integral to the wellbeing of the neurodivergent individual.

Each member of a neurodivergent person's support team fulfils a specific and valuable role, the general features of which are outlined below:

Parents

For children and adolescents, parent(s) / primary caregivers are the most important people in the support team.[4] The role of the parents is, above all else, to provide love, acceptance, and security. Parents benefit from education around attachment (e.g., Circle of Security) adapted to accommodate the individual and neurological differences of their child. Parents also need access to high quality information and advice regarding their child's needs according to their individual profile. This may be provided by the relevant professionals on the team, but may also be sourced online, or through books, face to face trainings, support groups, or anywhere else one finds information. Most parents also benefit from their own therapy, primarily for assistance coping with the stress inherent in parenting alongside the additional demands of meeting the unique needs of their child.

The proverbial village

The proverb 'it takes a village to raise a child' speaks to the need for a community of many people to provide a safe and

---

[4]   In the interests of brevity 'parents' will be the term used to refer to a child's primary caregiver(s), irrespective of biological relationship. Primary caregivers may include adoptive, foster, or kinship carers, or other form of appointed legal guardian.

nourishing environment for a child, where they are given the security and breadth of experience they need to truly flourish. This is true for *all* children regardless of neurotype, but possibly more so for neurodivergent children, for a variety of reasons. Some parents are fortunate to have a natural 'village' of extended family and/or friends around them to lend an ear and a hand when needed, but many parents find themselves isolated, often with damaging effects. While public policy does afford some parents opportunities for establishing social connections, those services can be difficult to access, and often fail to meet the complex needs of neurodivergent families. Grassroots organisations providing support, information, and activities often serve as a village for folk who are fortunate enough to belong to such a community. However, there is a very real need for wide-spread organised, cohesive, quality, community-based supports to meet the need of families who find themselves isolated and struggling.

The professional team

Most children who are identified as autistic will engage with professionals whose role it is to offer skills relevant to their training with the aim of ensuring quality of life for the child and, by extension, their family. Many autistic folk will remain engaged with professionals (though perhaps not the same ones) into adolescence, and some into adulthood. For parents just starting out and trying to navigate the complex world of services and supports, a description of the role fulfilled by each profession may be helpful:

Educators

The core role of educators is to provide academic instruction, however by virtue of the sheer amount of time children spend at school, educators are also charged with providing social guidance, emotional support, and often behaviour management. With such multifaceted responsibilities, educators play a central role in the lives of children. For autistic students who find it difficult to connect with peers, teaching staff may be the only source of genuine human connection and comfort in what is often experienced as a demanding and overwhelming environment, and many neurodivergent students become deeply attached to the educators in their lives.

As a diagnostician I find the observations and insights of educators invaluable; they get to see how children navigate complex social situations, how they cope with demands, and how they learn. Educators are also in a unique position in that they observe the child within a group of same-aged peers, which is often when developmental differences become most apparent. In my experience, educators are often the most important members of a child's support team, after parents. For all these reasons, it is vitally important that each new teacher is informed about a child's individual differences and support needs, to allow them to provide the adjustments and accommodations necessary for the child to experience the classroom as a safe space, and to succeed as a learner.

Support worker (paid carer)

The core role of a support worker is to support their client
in activities of daily living, and to help them to achieve their
goals by providing both practical and emotional support.
The specific duties and responsibilities of a support worker
will vary significantly depending on the needs and wishes
of the client. For many autistic adults support workers
are essential to living a full and meaningful life, helping
with day-to-day tasks, facilitating social participation, and
providing companionship. For those folk fortunate enough
to have a skilled professional caregiver with whom they have
developed a trusting working alliance, the importance of
that worker as a member of the individual's support team
cannot be overstated.

Psychologist

As it is my own profession, I know more about the role of a
psychologist than I do any other. That said, my experience
is that of a clinical psychologist working in private practice,
and is quite different from the role of a psychologist with
different training, and/or experience working in a different
context. Indeed, most health professions are very varied, so
it pays to ask about the specific interests and expertise of a
professional you are considering engaging. Regardless, the
core role of a psychologist is to diagnose and treat psychiatric
illnesses. Many psychologists undertake additional training
to become proficient in identifying neurodevelopmental
differences through observational assessment, and by
systematically gathering information from the individual

and those directly involved in their life (i.e., parents, extended family members, educators, other professionals). Often an autism assessment results in identification of autism as well as diagnosis of one or more co-occurring conditions (i.e., depression, anxiety, PTSD, ADHD), as co-occurring conditions are the rule, rather than the exception, for neurodivergent folk. Beyond the assessment, a psychologist's role is to provide clients and their family with psycho-education (i.e., accurate information about autism and/or co-occurring conditions), recommendations for supports, and ongoing therapy as needed. In my experience, some newly identified neurodivergent folk need very little support beyond the initial development and implementation of a support plan. Other folk, often those with co-occurring mental health diagnoses, or the more nebulous 'autistic burnout', benefit from a course of therapy to help them restore wellbeing and develop a sustainable self-care regime.

Speech Pathologist

The core role of a speech pathologist is to diagnose and treat communication disorders, including difficulties with speaking, listening, understanding language, reading, writing, stuttering, and using voice. Speech pathologists are often involved in the process of assessing for autism and are an essential member in the therapeutic team for autistic people who have communication difficulties. For minimally verbal or non-speaking autistic folk, access to effective communication aides is facilitated by their speech pathologist. Speech pathologists also help people who experience difficulties with eating and drinking for sensory, physical, neurological, or mental health reasons.

Occupational Therapist

The core role of an occupational therapist is to support health and wellbeing by enabling people to participate in the everyday activities of daily living, such as self-care activities (i.e., showering, dressing, preparing food), productive activities (i.e., education, work, volunteering and caring for others), and leisure/social activities (i.e., being part of a community or friendship group, engaging in a hobby). Occupational therapists are often involved in the process of assessing for autism, in which their role is to assess the individual's functional ability across a variety of activities and settings, including the home, school, work, and social environments. Occupational therapists play a vital role in helping autistic folk to identify and implement the supports that facilitate participation in activities of daily living. Occupational therapists are trained to evaluate sensory processing and integrate sensory strategies into support plans to help people with sensory differences participate in the activities that are important to them.

Physiotherapist

The core role of a physiotherapist is to treat muscle, nerve, and joint problems. Physiotherapists often work with autistic children to help develop muscle tone, motor skills, improve balance and coordination, and help with posture and alignment. Physiotherapy may help with simple skills such as sitting and standing, as well as more complex skills such as playing, kicking, throwing, and catching. The goal of physiotherapy is often to for the client to be able to move more freely, and to be physically independent.

Dietitian

Dietitians are experts in food and nutrition, and their core role is to provide dietary guidance. For autistic folk whose food intake is impacted by sensory differences, strong food preferences, eating disorders, and feeding disorders, a dietitian experienced in working with neurodivergent clients can play an important role in their support team. Given the complexities inherent in eating and feeding difficulties in autistic people, relevant training and experience, along with a flexible approach, is essential.

Paediatrician

Paediatricians are medical specialists who diagnose, treat, and provide medical care for infants, children, and teenagers. A paediatrician is often the first port of call for parents with concerns about their child's development, and they are often involved in the process of assessing for autism. Beyond diagnosis, a paediatrician may prescribe medication to help with co-occurring conditions such as ADHD, anxiety, and depression, as well as treat any medical issues that are beyond the scope of a general practitioner.

Psychiatrist

Psychiatrists are medical specialists who diagnose and treat people with psychiatric conditions (i.e., anxiety, depression, bipolar disorder, schizophrenia) and neurodevelopmental differences that are treated with medication (e.g., ADHD). Some autistic folk may never need the input of a psychiatrist, however for those with co-occurring ADHD or mental health concerns such as anxiety or depression, a psychiatrist plays a vital role in their wellbeing, overseeing the medication management of symptoms.

Choosing team members

In an ideal world autistic folk and their families would be able to choose from a selection of suitably trained professionals, opting for the professionals they believed to be the best fit for their needs. Unfortunately, the reality is that, in most locations, there are relatively few suitably trained professionals, many of whom have very limited capacity for new clients. Faced with long waitlists, people understandably often accept the first offer of help without necessarily considering whether the skill set, approach, and personality of the professional in question is well suited to the needs of the person receiving their service. In the absence of a readily available solution for this pervasive problem, the invitation to those seeking professional support is to (a) ask potential providers one or more of the questions listed in Appendix A to gauge the extent to which their approach is neurodiversity affirming, (b) offer relevant educational materials, such as this book, and (c) trust your intuition with regard to the people you invite into your own or your child's life.

Communication between team members

Interprofessional collaboration is widely considered best practice, and is invaluable when well-coordinated, however in reality anything more than the requisite brief written correspondence between health care professionals is often a difficult goal to attain. Many professionals have full schedules, and coordinating a team of multiple professionals to be available at the same time for a stakeholder meeting can be near impossible, especially at short notice. Working within the aforementioned limitations, my recommendation is for, at minimum, a twice-yearly stakeholder meeting to share relevant information and insights, review progress, set person-centred goals for the months ahead, and identify any issues that need to be addressed. Planning the meeting to be around the same times each year, and scheduling it in well in advance, means that collaboration becomes a reality rather than an aspiration.

The therapeutic relationship

Note: it is my firm belief that all relationships have the potential to be therapeutic, regardless of professional training and role. Whether your role is that of a health professional, educator, support worker, or unpaid caregiver, the following principles are applicable, though the way in which they are expressed and/or demonstrated will vary depending on the context and nature of your relationship with the neurodivergent person. In the interest of clarity, I have presented the information within the frame of the therapist – client relationship.

Many neurodivergent folk, children and adolescents in particular, are engaged in multiple therapies on a long-term basis. By virtue of the sheer amount of time spent with therapists, along with the nature of the work that is done in therapy, the relationship between therapist and client has the potential to be a source of great support, and simultaneously has the potential to be a source of harm. The invitation is for therapists to prioritise the therapeutic relationship over all else. Expertise is redundant if the client does not feel safe, seen, accepted, and valued. The role of therapist is to hold a safe and nourishing space, remain curious and present, and to offer their skilled guidance where appropriate. The content of therapy sessions will be different for each discipline, however the importance of providing an emotionally safe container for the client to do their work is equally relevant to all therapists.

> "Loving Presence is a practice of ... simply being with another, human to human. It requires ... that we learn about our own habits and automatic tendencies, and decide whether they support or interfere with being present in this way. These might be habits of making assumptions, focusing on what (we perceive) is wrong, over-analysing, wanting or needing to fix, being impatient or busy trying to make something happen... The practice of Loving

Presence is great for therapists, but it is really for anyone. Learning even a little bit of this approach will make all of us more skillfully helpful... We can be helpful as friends or teachers, as parents or partners, as well as helping professionals." (Kurtz, 2019, pp. 19-20)

Below are some key considerations for creating an emotionally and physically safe environment. It is by no means and exhaustive list. Rather, it is a summary of the essential features of a neurodiversity affirming practice and/ or practitioner.

Presume Competence

To presume competence is to assume someone has the capacity to think, learn, and understand. In the absence of tangible evidence one way or the other, presuming competence is the least dangerous assumption; should the initial assumption prove to be wrong an assumption of competence stands to do less harm to the individual than an assumption of incompetence (Donnellan, 1984). This is particularly relevant for minimally verbal autistic folk. Many people incorrectly associated the absence of speech with low intelligence, however in as many as 50 percent of minimally verbal autistics this is not the case (Bal, 2016), and given the right supports these folk often demonstrate competence that is average or above.

Informed consent

All appropriately trained health care professionals have a process in place to gain informed consent before working with a client. During this process the nature of the service to be provided is explained, and the client confirms they understand and are participating voluntarily, often by signing a form at the beginning of the first consult. The manner and frequency with which the clinician approaches the matter of informed consent tends to depend on their individual style and organisational policy. In my experience the best processes for gaining informed consent from neurodivergent clients share the following features:

1. Delivery of information uses plain language, is multimodal (i.e., verbal, written, and visual), and provisions are available to accommodate any communication differences (i.e., communication aides such as assistive technology are made available and used effectively).

2. Clients are afforded as much time as they need to process the information before providing consent. This may mean providing links to information by email prior to the initial consult.

3. Clients are explicitly provided with the opportunity to ask questions at the time of providing consent, as well as an invitation to ask questions at any time throughout the therapeutic relationship.

4. Each session starts with an outline of the therapist's proposed session plan (assuming one exists), and a

check-in to confirm the client consents, as well as to ask the client what is most important for them to talk about that day[5].

5. For therapists who use touch (i.e., physiotherapists, speech pathologists, occupational therapists) it is essential to ask for consent every time physical contact is necessary, and to inform the client exactly what the physical contact will involve before proceeding.

Informed consent for vulnerable clients

There are additional layers to the process of gaining informed consent when the client is a child or adolescent under the age of sixteen. Though many older children and young adolescents can make day to day decisions for themselves, many cannot, and legally all minors lack capacity to provide informed consent for healthcare procedures by virtue of their age alone. When working with minors the clinician must gain the informed consent of parents, as well as confirm with the child that they are a willing participant, generally referred to as gaining *assent*.

My approach is to convey to the child, using whatever language is best suited to their age and level of understanding, that I am first and foremost an ally and advocate, and secondary to that my role is to be a mentor or teacher, and sometimes a translator between the child and the adults in

---

[5]   In my experience, client's often come to session with something specific they want to work on, in which case my plan is shelved, and we focus on the topic chosen by the client.

their lives. My style is play-informed, and my therapy space is set up to be very child friendly, with games, toys, drums and other percussion instruments, a sweet little therapy dog and a virtual reality headset with biofeedback training. Parents are often present in sessions, but when I work one to one with children, I offer confidentiality because I see the benefit in having a safe and private space to talk, though I do make clear from the outset that risk of harm negates confidentiality. I do this by stating to both parents and child that if there is anything that causes me to feel worried about the child, I will let the child know first, and together we will make a plan for talking to the parents and/or the relevant adult(s). I also check in regularly by inviting the child to ask me anything at all they might be wondering about. I do occasionally get asked some odd and/or personal questions, but generally children ask questions that are relevant to therapy and helpful to them, and I find the simple act of being open to sharing about myself is a reliable way to establish trust and transparency with children. To date, I have never needed to decline to answer a question because it was too personal or inappropriate, though I do have a kind and gentle response prepared just in case.

Similarly, it is necessary to exercise caution when working with adults with intellectual disability, many of whom are, ethically and legally, considered to have limited capacity to provide informed consent. Often, but not always, there is a legal guardian who will first provide consent, and the same principles apply in terms of gaining informed consent /

assent from the client. The focus is around ensuring clarity and appropriateness of communication, providing the client with ample time to consider what is being proposed, explicitly inviting questions, and regularly checking in to confirm the client's assent is ongoing. The means by which these steps are achieved will be guided by the individual needs of the client, and professional training and supervision is recommended for clinicians entering this space.

Therapeutic Goals

Communication between therapist and client is an essential pre-requisite to developing therapeutic goals. For clients who do not have a robust and effective method of communication, facilitating access to a speech pathologist who can provide appropriate supports is the priority. Supports may include therapy to develop speech and language skills and/or assistance to effectively use Augmentative and Alternative Communication (AAC). Once an effective mode of communication has been established the client should be directly involved in all goal setting and support planning. Affirming goals are person-centred, meaning that they are centred around, and work towards the wishes, hopes, and aspirations of the client. Neurodiversity affirming services aim to eliminate barriers that preventing the individual from achieving their goals, and support the individual to develop necessary skills, or address specific problems. Most notably, reducing the outward appearance of autistic traits is not an acceptable target for intervention. Rather, intervention targets must directly relate to a person-centred goal with the aim of improving subjective quality of life, and be explicitly agreed to by the autistic person (ASAN).

Ableism in Language

Many readers will be familiar with the term 'ableism', however my experience leads me to believe there will be some who are not, so a definition and brief explanation seems appropriate. Ableism is a form of discrimination and prejudice against people with disabilities, or those who are perceived as having disabilities. It involves the belief that people with disabilities are inferior, or less valuable than those without disabilities. An ableist society is one that treats non-disabled people as the 'standard' of normal living. Often, this results in public places and services being designed to cater for the 'standard' majority, without making adjustments for people with 'non-standard' experiences.

Ableism can manifest in various forms, such as physical or social barriers that limit access to education, employment, housing, and other opportunities. Ableism is also present in negative stereotypes and attitudes towards people with disabilities, such as assuming that they are less intelligent, less competent, less capable of having rewarding relationships, or less deserving of respect. Ableism can be both intentional and unintentional, and exists at an individual level, an institutional level, and a cultural level. Ableism has significant negative impacts on the lives of people with disabilities, limiting opportunities, causing emotional distress, and leading to social isolation.

A commitment to neurodiversity affirming practice requires the practitioner to develop awareness around the dynamics of privilege and oppression in general, and ableism, specifically, and to engage in regular self-reflection. For folk approaching this work from a position of relative privilege, developing a deep understanding and awareness of the many facets of privilege and ableism may take time; the invitation is to maintain an open, curious mind, and to hold yourself and others with compassion.

Ableism lies hidden in the most obvious places, and nowhere is more pervasive than in our language. Below are some suggestions for simple but powerful changes. These are what I would consider the basic requirements of affirming care.

1. Replace 'disorder' with 'difference'. In the Diagnostic and Statistical Manual (DSM) every diagnostic label ends with the word 'disorder' (i.e., autism spectrum disorder, major depressive disorder, generalised anxiety disorder), and this is unlikely to change any time soon. However, by replacing the word 'disorder' with 'difference' in everyday speech and written communication, the autistic community and its supporters are effectively rejecting pathologizing labels and reclaiming autism as a valued identity.

2. Ask autistic folk how they would like to be referred to. The general community consensus is a preference for identity first language. That means saying 'autistic person', rather than using person-first terms such as 'person with autism', or 'person on the spectrum'. Proponents of person first language, generally not autistic folk themselves, argue that it serves to acknowledge the person as separate from

their disability. However, autism is integral to the lives and identities of autistic folk, and not something that can be compartmentalised away. Artificially distancing a person's disability from their humanity is potentially harmful. That said, there a there are certainly folk with different opinions on the matter, and my firm belief is that it is always better to ask than to assume.

3. Avoid using the terms 'high functioning' and 'low functioning'. These terms are misleading at best (i.e., an autistic person may outwardly appear to be functioning at a high level, yet their internal experience may be one of complete overwhelm and distress), and derogatory at worst. Current best practice is to refer to individual differences in ability in terms of 'support needs'. As mentioned previously, support needs, as described by the DSM, include level 1 (requiring support), level 2 (requiring substantial support), and level 3 (requiring very substantial support), however when used out of context, levels may also be misleading. The reality is that support needs are dynamic, changing in response to factors both within and around the autistic person, and across the lifespan. That said, 'support needs' is still the most widely accepted and affirming terminology.

4. Replace 'comorbid' with co-occurring'. The term 'comorbid' specifically relates to diseases or medical conditions. As autism is a neurotype rather than a disease, the accurate term for different neurodevelopmental or mental health diagnoses that exist alongside autism is 'co-occurring conditions'.

Cultural humility

Cultural humility is a core characteristic of a neurodiversity affirming therapists. The neurodiversity movement encourages us to understand neurodivergence from a cultural perspective, whereby neurodiversity is a culture with membership of people with diagnosed or self-identified neurodivergence, commonly autism and ADHD, and inclusive of a wide range of brain-based human differences. Neurodiversity culture encompasses all the knowledge and values shared by the neurodivergent community, preferred methods of expression and communication, and representative art and literature (Gobbo, 2019). For the neurodiversity affirming therapist, cultural humility is a commitment to the lifelong process of self-reflection and self-critique whereby we examine our own beliefs, assumptions, biases, and values, explore how our background and social context has shaped our understanding of neurodiversity as a culture (Yeager, 2013). Though the starting points may vary, cultural humility is equally relevant for neurodivergent and neurotypical therapists, as we all potentially bring unconscious biases into our practice.

The physical environment

The environment in which therapy takes place is important when supporting neurodivergent clients. Universal design is an approach to creating environments, products, and services that are inclusive and accessible for all people, including neurodivergent folk. The goal is to design and create spaces, products, and services that are flexible, easy to use, and accommodate a wide range of abilities. It aims to provide support and accommodations for autistic folk in a way that is integrated, rather than segregated, into the design of the environment. For a comprehensive checklist of accessibility considerations visit: http://www.stopableism. org/p/accessible-businesses.

Recommended adjustments include:

- Clear and consistent signage and labelling in buildings, so people can easily navigate their surroundings.

- Providing visual schedules, social stories, and other visual aids to help people understand expectations and routines.

- Flexible seating options, so that people can choose their preferred seating arrangements.

- Providing sensory-friendly spaces, such as quiet rooms, areas with low lighting, or a fragrance-free zone for people who may be sensitive to certain stimuli.

- Using simple, clear language, to ensure that information is easily understood.

- Involve neurodivergent people and their families in the design process to ensure that their needs and perspectives are considered.

Personally, I have a deep appreciation for comfort and aesthetics, as well as a few sensory sensitivities, so creating a therapy space that is calm, inviting, and comfortable has always been a high priority for me. Below are some of the additional adjustments I have found helpful:

1. Incorporate natural light, and avoid fluorescent light where possible. When choosing artificial lights, opt for a combination of lamps and overhead lights with dimmer switches. Invite clients to choose lighting that suits their preference.

2. Keep a selection of cushions, weighted blankets and plushies, sensory items, and fidget toys accessible. Moreover, making use of such items yourself gives clients authentic permission to do the same.

3. Have a standing invitation for clients to 'come as you are'. Explicitly invite clients to unmask. Unmasking may mean stimming, bringing comfort items from home, not making eye contact, and any number of behaviours that help the person regulate.

The importance of resolving ruptures in the therapeutic relationship

The neurodiversity paradigm is relatively new to the mainstream, and the neurodiversity affirming approach to care is newer still. For many clinicians and helping professionals, the shift to an affirming approach means unlearning much of what was explicitly taught and/or implied throughout our professional training. As such, it is essential that we are conscientious, intentional, reflective, humble, and compassionate towards our clients and ourselves. There is genuine value in undergoing professional development, engaging in regular peer supervision, and keeping abreast of current literature. However, even for those clinicians who consider themselves well informed, mistakes will happen. For some clients, the mistake will be experienced as harmful, and in those cases will likely result in a rupture in the therapeutic relationship. It is the job of the therapist to detect and address ruptures. When acknowledged and attended to, most mistakes can be corrected and most harm can be repaired.

Regardless of whether the rupture has been explicitly acknowledged by the client, it is important that a repair be instigated by the therapist. The following is a logical and empirically supported (Stolorow, 2000) process for repairing after a rupture.

1. Acknowledge the mistake.

2. Explain how and/or why the mistake happened. Help the client understand your motivation and intention.

3. Apologise.

4. Explain what you have learned, and what you will do differently in future as a result of that learning.

5. Ask what can be done to repair the relationship. Provide the client with time to consider their response and be open to communication in whatever form is most comfortable for the client.

In my experience as a budding psychologist, I found that mistakes tended to happen when I was feeling unsure. The dreaded imposter syndrome led me to feel compelled to *do something*. In doing something to ease my own discomfort, rather than because the client had guided the process, I risked alienating the client by clumsily positioning myself as the expert. It is true that clinicians bring a valuable skillset to the table, and certainly possession of suitable skills is an essential quality in a therapist, however knowing when and how to use that skill is paramount. The therapeutic relationship is a working alliance in which the client is ultimately the expert in their own life, and the therapist is a resource whose role is to support self-healing and growth within the client. It is a person-to-person relationship, and is ideally characterised by mutuality, transparency, respect, and authenticity. This is especially important when supporting neurodivergent folk, many of whom are highly sensitive to perceived rejection, and are likely to (quite reasonably) experience unsolicited advice as criticism. When in doubt, pause, breathe, and come back to the core values of respect, unconditional positive regard, and compassion for both client and self.

Trauma Informed Care

For people existing within environments and systems set up to cater for a neurotype other than their own, many events experienced as benign by neurotypical folk are experienced as overwhelming and potentially traumatic by neurodivergent folk. There is also ample evidence to indicate that neurodivergent folk are more likely to experience overt exclusion, maltreatment, and victimisation (Weiss, 2018). Add neurobiological differences that increase vulnerability to traumatic stress (Parellada, 2014), and the recommendation for trauma-informed care as standard practice needs no further justification.

Five core principles guide trauma informed care:

1. Safety. Steps are taken to ensure supports are experienced as emotionally and physically safe. Consideration is given to individual differences and needs (i.e., communication style, sensory sensitivities).

2. Trustworthiness and transparency. Care is sensitive to the needs of the individual, and decisions are made with transparency, and with the goal of building and maintaining trust.

3. Peer Support. The voices of people with shared lived experience are elevated and valued, and form an integral part of service delivery.

4. Choice and collaboration. Service provision is person-centred and supports shared decision making, with ultimate choice and control in the hands of the neurodivergent person.

5. Humility and Responsiveness. Trauma informed care recognises and addresses biases, stereotypes, and historical trauma.

Everyone who provides services to neurodivergent folk, most notably medical professionals, allied health professionals, education providers, and disability support workers, should undergo, at minimum, basic training in the presentations of anxiety and trauma in neurodivergent folk, and trauma-informed practices. The reasons for this are two-fold. Firstly, many behaviours that are traditionally viewed as 'challenging' are, in fact, reflective of an overwhelmed nervous system, while many of the traditional approaches to addressing 'challenging behaviours' fail to acknowledge this underlying need, and respond in ways that are further traumatising for the neurodivergent person. Second, a trauma informed approach to care acknowledges the increased likelihood that a neurodivergent person may have experienced trauma and takes steps to minimise the risk of further harm. Blue Knot Foundation, an Australian organisation catering to victims of complex trauma, provide some excellent free resources and paid training for those interested (see https://blueknot. org.au).

6. ROOF

Self-advocacy – the ability to communicate one's wants, needs, and opinions – is a vital life skill for neurodivergent folk. Effective self-advocacy requires that the neurodivergent person understands that there are people, systems, and legislation in place to support them, and knows who to approach for support. The roof refers to the people, systems, and legislation whose role it is to protect the rights of the neurodivergent person.

People

An advocate is any person who works to promote the rights and improve the quality of life of people with disabilities. At an individual level, any member of a neurodivergent person's team may act in an advocacy role. This may include providing information and resources, advocating for the recommended supports and accommodations to be implemented, and highlighting policies or practices that discriminate against the neurodivergent person. An advocate may also help the individual navigate the healthcare and social service systems, and to secure the support they need to live independently. Where additional help is required, engaging a disability advocacy service is recommended. In Australia, these are:

- The Disability Advocacy Finder: This is a service provided by the Australian government that helps people find advocacy services in their local area. https://askizzy. org.au/disability-advocacy-finder
- The Disability Advocacy Resource Unit (DARU): This is an organisation that provides support and resources to disability advocacy groups and individual advocates across Australia. https://www.daru.org.au
- People with Disability Australia (PWDA): This is a national disability rights and advocacy organisation that works to promote the rights and interests of people with disabilities, including autistic folk. https://pwd.org.au
- National Disability Services (NDS): This is the peak body for non-government disability service organisations in Australia. NDS provides a range of services and support to member organisations, including advocacy and representation at a national level. https://www.nds.org.au
- Council on Intellectual Disability (CID): This is a peak body that advocates for the rights of people with intellectual disability and their families and carers. https://cid.org.au

Systems

The systems in place to support and protect neurodivergent folk vary from location to location. In Australia the government funds the National Disability Insurance Scheme (NDIS), which aims to provide people with disabilities with access to the support they need to live independently and participate fully in their communities. This includes funding for disability-related services such as assistive technology, assistance with daily living, home modifications, and access to community activities. The NDIS aims to provide a system of support that is person-centred, flexible, and responsive to the unique needs of people with disabilities, empowering participants by giving them greater choice and control over the support services they receive. There are protective safeguards built into the Scheme whereby participants and/or their advocates can have concerns and issues addressed. As is often the case with large-scale government programs, the NDIS can be a difficult landscape to navigate, and many neurodivergent people benefit from the support of an advocate when accessing the scheme.

Legislation

Again, legislation varies from location to location. In Australia, the Disability Discrimination Act 1992 (DDA) and the Disability Standards for Education 2005 (DSE) protect the rights of people with disabilities. The DDA makes it unlawful to discriminate against a person on the basis of their disability in areas such as employment, education, and access to goods and services. The DSE sets out specific standards to ensure that students with disabilities, including autism, have equal access to education. Many organisations develop their policies and procedures with relevant legislation in mind, however this is not always the case, and there are certainly times when, for a range of reasons, there is a gap between policy and practice. At such times an advocate may be required to help the neurodivergent person have their concerns addressed.

7. WINDOW

The window refers to the lens through which the autistic person's behaviour is viewed, and the interpretations and responses that follow. The term 'challenging behaviour' has long been used to describe any behaviour that is difficult for the autistic person or the people around them. This typically includes behaviours such as aggression, self-injury, property destruction, and 'non-compliance'. It may also include behaviours that are core features of autism, such as stimming, difficulty with transitions, or avoidance social interactions. Being labelled as an autistic person with 'challenging behaviours' can make it difficult to access some educational and social opportunities, and can lead to exclusion from mainstream settings, without necessarily examining or explaining the context within which the behaviours arise.

The practice of viewing behaviour as communication means asking the following questions:

What does the behaviour tell us about the person's emotional experience?

- Uncertainty or fear: are they feeling uncertain or scared about what is being asked of them?
- Overwhelm: are the demands of the situation (i.e., sensory, cognitive, language, social) beyond their capacity to cope?
- Frustration: does the person not yet have the skills required to successfully navigate the situation? Is some aspect of the situation unjust, or otherwise frustrating for the person?
- Excitement: is the situation positive, but so much so that the emotion has become overwhelming?

What need is the person attempting to meet by engaging in the behaviour?

- Escape: do they need to withdraw from an activity or environment they experience as unpleasant or aversive?
- Respect: do they need to assert an interpersonal boundary?
- Space: do they need physical space?
- Understanding: do they need help with communication?

What support can be provided?

- Co-regulation: is there a trusted person who can help?
- Self-regulation: is there a space and/or tools available that will help the person to self-regulate?

- Communication: are there people or communication aides available to help the person communicate their needs effectively?

- Choice and control: is the person being supported to access what they want and need?

- Advocacy: does the person need someone to advocate for them in this situation? If so, who is the best person to do this?

A neuroscience-based perspective

The neuroscience approach to autism emphasises the importance of understanding the underlying neural mechanisms that drive behaviour, and incorporates research and knowledge from the field of neuroscience to understand how the brain functions differently in autistic people. Research using brain imaging has shown that autistic people have differences in brain structure and function compared to their typically developing peers (Ha, 2015). In particular, studies have shown differences in the form and function of the brain regions involved in the processing of social and emotional information (Kim S. C., 2015), and in the regulation of emotions such as fear and anxiety. These differences are thought to underlie differences in social behaviour, as well as increased anxiety and emotional reactivity among autistic folk (Hessl, 2022).

Studies have also shown differences in the structure and function of the brain regions involved in regulating attention (Rahko, 2016), which is thought to be related to the high rate of co-occurring ADHD (Christakou, 2013), as well as differences in the systems responsible for impulse control, which likely underlie repetitive behavioural traits (Mosconi, 2009). Additionally, differences the way brain regions communicate with each other have been observed in the language and imagery centres of the brain, which may explain why many autistic folk benefit from the use of visuals to support language comprehension (Kana, 2006).

The neuroscience of autism is a relatively recent and rapidly developing area of research. The brain is a highly complex organ and there is still much to learn, so while a neuroscience perspective can provide valuable insights into the underlying neural mechanisms that drive behaviour, it must be integrated with the following perspectives to truly be useful:

- Developmental perspective: this considers the unique developmental trajectory of the individual, and the relationship between their developmental stage and their behaviour.

- Ecological perspective: this considers how the individual interacts with their environment, including social and physical factors that may impact their behaviour.

- Cultural perspective: this considers how cultural and societal factors shape the understanding and support provided to autistic folk.

Most importantly, neuroscience research findings should not be used to pathologise or stereotype autism, only to provide a deeper understanding of the unique needs of each individual, and to develop more individualised and effective supports.

8. DOOR

The door refers to the ways in which the person connects with others, with emphasis on their *preferred* methods of connection. Many neurodivergent people are perfectly capable of connecting with others in all the usual neurotypical ways, but tend to find everyday interactions draining, and get the most enjoyment out of connection that fulfils certain neurodivergent needs. Others may require specific adjustments, such as assistive technology for communication, or may find some behaviours stressful, such as physical touch or eye contact. For some folk the simplest way to find out what their preferences are is to ask, however others may need help identifying what means of connection are most suited to their individual profile and needs. In all cases, the principles of informed consent, presuming competence, and cultural humility should remain central in all therapeutic relationships. Below are some features to consider:

- Communication: Does the person use language? Do they need or benefit from visual aides or other forms of assistive technology? Are they more comfortable with texting than phone calls? Do they pick up on subtext, or do they need explicit communication? Do they understand and/or enjoy indirect communication such as metaphor, sarcasm, and irony?

- Touch: how does the person feel about physical proximity and/or contact? What is the size of their personal space 'bubble'? What type of touch do they prefer, if any? When is touch not appropriate for them?

- Sensory: are there differences in the persons sensory profile which influence how they prefer to connect with others? Sensory sensitivities such as auditory and olfactory sensitivities are common, and impact factors such as choice of meeting place, and decision making around whether to wear perfume or cologne.

- Special interests: Most humans, regardless of neurotype, find it easier to connect with people who share similar interests. For neurodivergent folk, sharing information about special interests is particularly powerful in terms of providing a foundation for connection. What are their interests? Is this an interest you share, or know something about?

- Social interaction style: In social contexts, does the person enjoy conversation, or do they prefer to spend time together engaged in a shared activity, or working on separate parallel activities?

9. LANDSCAPE

The landscape refers to the socio-political environment in which the neurodivergent person lives, learns, works, and plays. I suspect most of my readers will have the good fortune to live in developed countries where quality research is funded, and the findings are (eventually) used to inform policy. These are mostly western, high-income countries; autism research is skewed for this reason. In fact, many of the 'gold-standard' diagnostic tools for autism were designed to be used with affluent, white, gender-conforming boys, and are of questionable value when used with people who deviate from this normative sample group (Langmann, 2017). We know less about the process of identifying and diagnosing autism in low- and middle-income settings, and how the experience of neurodivergent folk varies across cultures and contexts (de Leeuw, 2020).

We do know that autistic folk from minority groups in high income countries are less likely to engage with services, receive a diagnosis, or access supports, the reasons for which are manifold and related to intersectionality (Samadi, 2022). We also know that disabled folk in developing countries are additionally disadvantaged in a range of ways, including being less likely to receive quality education, less likely to attain employment, more likely to be a victim of violence, and having limited access to healthcare and supports (UNESCO, 2022). It is therefore crucial that the landscape is taken into taken into account when considering how best to build an affirming support network for, or as, a neurodivergent person.

Questions to ask:

1. What policies can be reviewed to better understand the systemic environment? Consider reading the inclusion policy, if one is available, for the person's specific school, the broader education system, and/or their employer. These are generally published on the organisation website. For example, Queensland Department of Education have published an Inclusive Education Policy which outlines the guiding principles which, to some extent, will shape the experience of all students with a diagnosed disability in Queensland State Schools (Education, 2021). Many schools and employers have a similar policy, and if not, the absence of such a policy is in and of itself informative. For organisations with an appropriate policy in place, the next question is whether the organisation has adequate resources to effectively implement the policy (i.e., do the staff have access to training, are there enough suitably trained staff, are there systems in place to monitor implementation of the policy)?

2. What are the local community's cultural values around diversity in general, and more specifically around

disability? Are community members from minority groups (i.e., ethnic, religious, sexuality, gender identity) welcomed and valued within the community? What about community members with visible disabilities (i.e., mobility challenges, vision and hearing impaired)? Are there supports available to ensure community spaces such as parks, shops, libraries, and entertainment facilities are accessible to all? What is the level of community awareness around neurodiversity? Is it a topic that is spoken about openly, or does a culture of secrecy and/or shame exist?

3. What information, services, and supports are available for neurodivergent folk, specifically? The internet means that most people are able to access information and online services with relative ease, whereas the availability of face-to-face services and supports vary considerably with location.

4. More importantly, is the information or service neurodiversity affirming? It can be difficult for people who are still learning about neurodiversity affirming care to know which information is reliable, and which services are worthy of their time and money. It is important to have a process for evaluation so as not to inadvertently take on misleading information, or engage a potentially unhelpful service. For example, a very prominent organisations in the autism space, often among the first listings on Google when searching 'what is autism', has received enormous criticism from the neurodivergent community for practices that perpetuate

stigma and create barriers to the inclusion of autistic people. Neurodiversity affirming service providers share the overarching values of individuality, choice, dignity, acceptance, respect, and collaboration. A checklist of potential questions to ask when evaluating a service providers is provided in Appendix A.

5. How accessible are the services that are available? This will be impacted by the socio-economic factors (i.e., what is the individual or family's level of education, income, and geographical location), systemic factors (i.e., is healthcare socialised or privatised), the ratio of healthcare providers to service users within the community, and the mode of delivery for services (i.e., is there flexibility in the delivery of services to accommodate the individual accessibility needs of service users?).

The socio-political landscape is often the last place change is seen, occurring once a 'tipping point' has been reached. The tipping point is the critical moment or threshold at which a collection of small changes or actions lead to a significant, and often irreversible outcome. It is the point at which a system or situation undergoes a rapid and dramatic transformation. The optimist in me sees reason to believe that we are approaching a tipping point with regard to embracing neurodiversity - a point at which the positive feedback loops begin to take hold, leading to a virtuous cycle of increasing awareness and acceptance. The realist in me sees the barriers and knows there is still a lot of work to be done.

What *can* be done?

- Join or form a coalition: By working together, people and organisations can leverage their collective resources, expertise, and influence to achieve greater impact than they could on their own. Coalitions can also help to build trust and relationships among diverse groups, encourage sharing of knowledge and skills, and increase the visibility and credibility of a cause or issue.

- Advocate for policy changes: Changing policies is one of the most direct ways to effect change in the socio-political landscape. This can involve lobbying, demonstrations, or using social media and other platforms to raise awareness of key issues.

- Promote education and awareness: By promoting understanding and knowledge of key issues, advocates and activists can help create a groundswell of public support for change.

- Support diverse leadership: Diversity in leadership is critical to changing the socio-political landscape. It is encouraging to see prominent people across all sectors disclosing their neurodivergence, and I love watching activists like Greta Thunberg and Grace Tame work. They are wonderful representatives and spokespeople for the neurodivergent community. We need many more neurodivergent people in positions of influence and leadership, and the support of the community is invaluable in helping to achieve this.

10. THE FUTURE

The lived experiences of neurodivergent folk in general, and autistic folk specifically, are varied and often complex. In a society that, by and large, caters to the neurotypical majority, neurodivergent folk often find themselves in the margins, perhaps due to their individual differences and needs, but more likely due to a failure of the systems and people around them to acknowledge and understand those needs, and to take meaningful steps to meet them. To Embrace Neurodiversity is to make a commitment to do what can be done to create environments in which neurodivergent people experience acceptance, understanding, and support. If enough people commit to Embracing Neurodiversity, the impairment so often caused by a mismatch between neurodivergent people and their environment will lessen, and a good many more people will come to see neurodiversity as something to be celebrated.

The Safe House Framework is one tool in the toolkit for people who know, love, work with, teach, or serve a neurodivergent human, and who want an approach that is both respectful and helpful. It is a way of organising one's thinking, and a guide for people who may not be sure which questions need to be asked, or who to approach for the answers. The Safe House is also a symbol, a way of communicating to the neurodivergent community that the individual or service is a neurodiversity ally, and committed to practices that are sensitive to the specific needs and abilities of neurodivergent folk.

At a broader level, the Safe House is a framework for thinking about how best to effect systemic change with the aim of reaching a point where society embraces neurodivergent minds, and seeks out the contributions of people who think and see things differently. Change of this magnitude will require collaboration and integration across education, health, legal, and government systems. In order for educational and therapeutic spaces to truly be a Safe House for neurodivergent folk, we need ongoing critical review of current evidence-based practices with direct input from the neurodivergent community, as well as widespread education (and re-education), and a steadfast commitment to continuous refinement of person-centred models of care.

Where to from here?

As a big-picture thinker, I have a clear vision for The Safe House Framework. As an autistic woman with some executive functioning differences, the steps required to bring the vision to life are less clear to me. I have decided to start with this book, and an accompanying online training program for professionals and parents of autistic children. I opted to start with children for two reasons. Firstly, it is the area of clinical practice in which

I have the most experience, which made it the simplest place to start. Secondly, human nature tends to make adults want to look after children; we recognise their innate vulnerability, and are drawn to protect them. This is obviously a broad generalisation, however it is the truth for many, and reason to think that The Safe House in its current form may be most readily adopted by the adults supporting autistic children.

The decision to group professionals and parents together was based on the belief that parents are the ultimate expert in their child, and charged with coordinating their child's professional supports. As such, it is imperative that parents and professionals are approaching the child's care from the same, neurodiversity affirming perspective. Beyond the initial training I will offer a Masterclass series for professionals, during which participants will be invited to deepen their knowledge of autism and neurodiversity affirming practice.

Part of my vision for The Safe House is a provider list of professionals who have completed the Masterclass series, and who have attained a high level of competence in all areas of Neurodiversity Affirming Practice. Such a list will provide neurodivergent people and their families a way to identify providers who are genuinely committed to the values of neurodiversity affirming practice, and have knowledge and practical skills to match. A similar training for professionals working with adult populations will follow.

To complement the training, I am working on an app to disseminate education related to neurodiversity affirming practice within multidisciplinary teams, and to support interdisciplinary communication and collaboration. The app, owned by the neurodivergent person, will host their Safe House Support Plan. The person and/or their representative will have the ability to grant access to members of their professional team so that they can view and contribute to the Support Plan, and to anyone providing supports (i.e., relatives, teachers, disability support workers).

Most of all, my hope is that society's understanding of neurodiversity, and acceptance of autistic folk, continues to grow. In some sections of society we have made very real progress, but we still have a long way to go before our autistic community members will feel safe to show up authentically in any context without fear of being met with stigma, fear, or rejection. The Safe House is a way to mark out safe territory for neurodivergent folk. The hope is that, as the number of Safe Houses grows, our communities will become more welcoming, supportive places for everyone.

Thank you for reading this far! If you would like to learn how to implement The Safe House in your life, home, classroom, or workplace, go to www.embracingneurodiversity.co/book and register to receive updates on training offerings.

If you found this book helpful, please share it with others who may also find it helpful.

BIBLIOGRAPHY

APA. (2022). *Diagnostic and Statistical Manual of Mental Disorders, 5th Edition, Text Revision.* American Psychiatric Association.

Arora, I. B. (2021). Is autonomic function during resting-state atypical in Autism: A systematic review of evidence. *Neuroscience & Biobehavioral Reviews., 125,* 417-441.

ASAN. (2022). *For Whose Benefit? Evidence, Ethics, and Effectiveness of Autism Interventions.* Retrieved from Autistic Self Advocacy Network: https://autisticadvocacy.org/wp-content/uploads/2021/12/ACES-Ethics-of-Intervention.pdf

Bal, V. H. (2016). Understanding definitions of minimally verbal across instruments: evidence for subgroups within minimally verbal children and adolescents with autism spectrum disorder. *. Journal of child psychology and psychiatry, and allied disciplines,* 1424-1433.

Banes, D. (2021, July 19). *Addressing Neurodiversity Through Universal Design.* Retrieved from Different Brains: https://differentbrains.org/addressing-neurodiversity-through-universal-design/

Baraskewich, J. v. (2021). Feeding and eating problems in children and adolescents with autism: A scoping review. *. Autism : the international journal of research and practice,* 1505–1519.

Baron-Cohen, S. W. (2001). "Reading the Mind in the Eyes" Test revised version: A study with normal adults, and adults with Asperger syndrome or high-functioning autism. *Journal of Child Psychology and Psychiatry,* 241-251.

Ben-Sasson, A. H.-Y. (2009). A meta-analysis of sensory modulation symptoms in individuals with autism spectrum disorders. *Journal of autism and developmental disorders*, 1-11.

Biggs, M. (2022). Suicide by Clinic-Referred Transgender Adolescents in the United Kingdom. *Archives of sexual behavior., 51*(2), 685–690.

Brewer, R. a. (2016, July 13). *People with Autism Can Read Emotions, Feel Empathy.* Retrieved from Scientific American: https://www.scientificamerican.com/article/people-with-autism-can-read-emotions-feel-empathy1/

Brown, T. (2006). Executive Functions and Attention Deficit Hyperactivity Disorder: Implications of two conflicting views. *International Journal of Disability Development and Education*, 35-45.

Cage, E. &.-W. (2019). Understanding the reasons, contexts and costs of camouflaging for autistic adults. *Journal of autism and developmental disorders*, 1899-1911.

Carmassi, C. P. (2019). Systematic Review of Sleep Disturbances and Circadian Sleep Desynchronization in Autism Spectrum Disorder: Toward an Integrative Model of a Self-Reinforcing Loop. *Frontiers in Psychiatry* .

Chapman, R. (2021). Neurodiversity and the Social Ecology of Mental Functions. *Perspectives on Psychological Science*.

Charman, T. P. (2011). IQ in children with autism spectrum disorders: Data from the Special Needs and Autism Project (SNAP). *Psychological Medicine*, 619-627.

Chown, N. B. (2017). Theoretical Models and Autism. In F. Volkmar, *Encyclopedia of Autism Spectrum Disorders*. New York, NY.: Springer.

Christakou, A. M. (2013). Disorder-specific functional abnormalities during sustained attention in youth with Attention Deficit

Hyperactivity Disorder (ADHD) and with autism. *Molecular psychiatry., 18*(2), 236-244.

Clapp, M. A. (2017). Gut microbiota's effect on mental health: The gut-brain axis. *Clinics and practice., 7*(4), 987.

Cohen, S. C. (2014). The relationship between sleep and behavior in autism spectrum disorder (ASD): a review. *Journal of Neurodevelopmental Disorders., 6*(44).

de Leeuw, A. H. (2020). A Conceptual Framework for Understanding the Cultural and Contextual Factors on Autism Across the Globe. *Autism Research,* 1029-1050.

Deliens, G. L. (2015). Sleep Disturbances in Autism Spectrum Disorders. *Review Journal of Autism and Developmental Disorders., 2,* 343–356.

Donnellan, A. (1984). The Criterion of the Least Dangerous Assumption. *Behavioral Disorders,* 141-150.

Education, Q. D. (2021, August 10). *Policy and Procedure Register.* Retrieved from Inclusive Education Policy: https://ppr.qed.qld. gov.au/pp/inclusive-education-policy

Fenning, R. M. (2019). Sympathetic-Parasympathetic Interaction and Externalizing Problems in Children with Autism Spectrum Disorder. . *Autism research : official journal of the International Society for Autism Research,* 1805-1816.

Gobbo, K. &. (2019). Should Neurodiversity Culture Influence How Instructors Teach? *Academic Exchange Quarterly.*

Ha, S. S. (2015). Characteristics of Brains in Autism Spectrum Disorder: Structure, Function and Connectivity across the Lifespan. *Experimental neurobiology., 24*(4), 273-284.

Hessl, D. L.-P. (2022). Fear Potentiated Startle in Children With Autism Spectrum Disorder: Association With Anxiety Symptoms and Amygdala Volume. *Autism research : official journal of the International Society for Autism Research., 14*(3), 450–463.

Hogan, A. (2019). Social and medical models of disability and mental health: evolution and renewal. *Canadian Medical Association Journal*, E16-E18.

Hours, C. R. (2022). ASD and ADHD Comorbidity: What Are We Talking About? *Frontiers in Psychiatry*.

Hull, L. P.-C. (2017). "Putting on My Best Normal": Social Camouflaging in Adults with Autism Spectrum Conditions. *Journal of autism and developmental disorders*, 2519-2534.

Johnson, K. (2020). Gut microbiome composition and diversity are related to human personality traits. *Human microbiome journal., 15*.

Kana, R. K. (2006). Sentence comprehension in autism: thinking in pictures with decreased functional connectivity. *Brain., 129*(9), 2484–2493.

Kang, D. W.-M.-B. (2019). Long-term benefit of Microbiota Transfer Therapy on autism symptoms and gut microbiota. *Scientific reports., 9*(1), 5821.

Kapp, S. (2019). *Autistic Community and the Neurodiversity Movement*. Singapore: Palgrave Macmillan .

Kaylene, G. (2022). *Autistic Mama*. Retrieved from 5 Important Reasons Even "New ABA" is Problematic: https://autisticmama.com/even-new-aba-is-problematic/

Kim, J. Y.-P. (2022). Association between autism spectrum disorder and inflammatory bowel disease: A systematic review and meta-analysis. *Autism research : official journal of the International Society for Autism Research., 15*(2), 340-352.

Kim, S. C. (2015). Abnormal activation of the social brain network in children with autism spectrum disorder: an FMRI study. *Psychiatry investigation., 12*(1), 37–45.

Koomar, T. T. (2021). Estimating the Prevalence and Genetic Risk Mechanisms of ARFID in a Large Autism Cohort. *Frontiers in Psychiatry., 12*.

Kurtz, R. &. (2019). *The Practice of Loving Presence: A Mindful Guide To Open-Hearted Relating.* Stone's Throw Publications.

Kurtz, R. &. (2019). *The Practice of Loving Presence: A Mindful Guide To Open-Hearted Relating.* Stones Throw Publications.

Lai, C. L. (2017). Meta-analysis of neuropsychological measures of executive functioning in children and adolescents with high-functioning autism spectrum disorder. *Autism Research,* 911-939.

Langmann, A. B.-B. (2017). Diagnostic utility of the autism diagnostic observation schedule in a clinical sample of adolescents and adults. *Research in Autism Spectrum Disorders,* 34-43.

Larsson, H. A. (2012). Childhood attention-deficit hyperactivity disorder as an extreme of a continuous trait: a quantitative genetic study of 8,500 twin pairs. *J Child Psychol Psychiatry.*

Leader, G. A. (2022). Gastrointestinal Symptoms in Autism Spectrum Disorder: A Systematic Review. *Nutrients.*

Leaf, J. B. (2022). Concerns About ABA-Based Intervention: An Evaluation and Recommendations. *Journal of autism and developmental disorders,* 2838-2853.

Lee, M. K.-G.-L. (2018). Association of Autism Spectrum Disorders and Inflammatory Bowel Disease. *Journal of autism and developmental disorders., 48*(5), 1523–1529.

Lovaas, O. K. (1973). Some generalization and follow-up measures on autistic children in behavior therapy. *. Journal of Applied Behavior Analysis.,* 131-165.

Ludyga, S. P. (2021). Muscle strength and executive function in children and adolescents with autism spectrum disorder. *Autism Research,* 2555– 2563.

Mannion, A. L. (2013). Sleep Problems in Autism Spectrum Disorder: A Literature Review. *Review Journal of Autism and Developmental Disorders., 1,* 101–109.

Mannion, A. L. (2014). Sleep Problems in Autism Spectrum Disorder: A Literature Review. *Review Journal of Autism and Developmental Disorders., 1*, 101-109.

Milton, D. (2012). On the ontological status of autism: the 'double empathy problem'. *Disability and Society*, 883-887.

Milton, D. (2019). *Damian Milton on Monotropism and Flow States*. Retrieved from Studio III Atlass: https://www.youtube.com/watch?v=MUDQD1p2zFE

Miyake, A. F. (2000). The unity and diversity of executive functions and their contributions to complex "Frontal Lobe" tasks: a latent variable analysis. *Cognitive psychology*, 49-100.

Monteiro, M. &. (2018). Monteiro interview guidelines for diagnosing the Autism Spectrum, Second Edition . Los Angeles, CA: Western Psychological Services.

Mosconi, M. W. (2009). Impaired inhibitory control is associated with higher-order repetitive behaviors in autism spectrum disorders. *Psychological medicine., 39*, 1559–1566.

Murray, D. L. (2005). Attention, monotropism and the diagnostic criteria for autism. *Autism*, 139-156.

O'Nions, E. G. (2016). Identifying features of 'pathological demand avoidance' using the Diagnostic Interview for Social and Communication Disorders (DISCO). *European Child & Adolescent Psychiatry., 25*, 407–419.

Oliver, M. (2013). The social model of disability: thirty years on. *Disability and Society*, 1024-10-26.

O'Nions, E. V. (2018). Dimensions of difficulty in children reported to have an autism spectrum diagnosis and features of extreme/'pathological' demand avoidance. *Child and Adolescent Mental Health., 23*, 220-227.

Ozsivadjian, A. (2020). Editorial: Demand avoidance — pathological, extreme or oppositional? *Child and Adolescent Mental Health., 25,* 57-58.

Parellada, M. P.-V. (2014). The neurobiology of autism spectrum disorders. *European Psychiatry,* 11-19.

Pearson, A. a. (2021). A Conceptual Analysis of Autistic Masking: Understanding the Narrative of Stigma and the Illusion of Choice . *Autism in Adulthood,* 52-60.

Pfeiffer, B. S. (2019). Effectiveness of Noise-Attenuating Headphones on Physiological Responses for Children With Autism Spectrum Disorders. *Frontiers in Integrative Neuroscience., 13.*

Postorino, V. K. (2017). Anxiety Disorders and Obsessive-Compulsive Disorder in Individuals with Autism Spectrum Disorder. . *Current Psychiatry Reports.*

Rahko, J. S.-G. (2016). Attention and working memory in adolescents with autism spectrum disorder: a functional MRI study. *Child Psychiatry & Human Development., 47,* 503 - 517.

Reynolds, A. M. (2019). Sleep Problems in 2- to 5-Year-Olds With Autism Spectrum Disorder and Other Developmental Delays. *Pediatrics., 143*(3).

Rossignol, D. &. (2011). Melatonin in autism spectrum disorders: a systematic review and meta-analysis. *Developmental Medicine and Child Neurology., 53*(9), 783-792.

Runswick-Cole, K. (2014). 'Us' and 'them': the limits and possibilities of a 'politics of neurodiversity' in neoliberal times. *Disability and Society,* 1117-1129.

Russell, G. (2020). Critiques of the Neurodiversity Movement. In S. Kapp, *Autistic Community and the Neurodiversity Movement* (pp. 287-303). Singapore: Palgrave Macmillan.

Rydzewska, E. H.-M. (2019). Prevalence of long-term health conditions in adults with autism: observational study of a whole country population. *British Medical Journal*, 819-829.

Samadi, S. A. (2022). Overview of Services for Autism Spectrum Disorders (ASD) in Low- and Middle-Income Countries (LMICs) and among Immigrants and Minority Groups in High-Income Countries (HICs). *Brain Sciences*, 1682.

Seif, A. S. (2021). A Systematic Review of Brainstem Contributions to Autism Spectrum Disorder. *Frontiers in Integrative Neuroscience.*, 15.

Singer, J. (2017). *NeuroDiversity: The Birth of and Idea.* Judy Singer.

Srikantha, P. &. (2019). The Possible Role of the Microbiota-Gut-Brain-Axis in Autism Spectrum Disorder. *International Journal of Molecular Sciences., 20*(9), 2115.

Steer, C. G. (2010). Traits contributing to the autistic spectrum. *PLoS One.*

Stolorow, R. B. (2000). *Psychoanalytic Treatment: An Intersubjective Approach.* California: Analytic Press.

Strang, J. F.-L.-L.-T. (2018). Revisiting the Link: Evidence of the Rates of Autism in Studies of Gender Diverse Individuals. *. Journal of the American Academy of Child and Adolescent Psychiatry*, 885–887.

Stuart, L. G. (2020). Intolerance of uncertainty and anxiety as explanatory frameworks for extreme demand avoidance in children and adolescents. *Child and Adolescent Mental Health.*, 25, 59-67.

Taniya, M. A. (2022). Role of Gut Microbiome in Autism Spectrum Disorder and Its Therapeutic Regulation. *Frontiers in cellular and infection microbiology.*

Taniya, M. A. (2022). Role of Gut Microbiome in Autism Spectrum Disorder and Its Therapeutic Regulation. *Frontiers in cellular and infection microbiology.*, 12.

Tordjman, S. N.-L. (2013). Advances in the research of melatonin in autism spectrum disorders: literature review and new perspectives. *International journal of molecular sciences., 14*(10), 20508–20542.

UNESCO. (2022, December 30). *United Nations* . Retrieved from Department of Economic and Social Affairs (Disability): https://www.un.org/development/desa/disabilities/resources/factsheet-on-persons-with-disabilities

Veatch, O. J. (2015). Genetic variation in melatonin pathway enzymes in children with autism spectrum disorder and comorbid sleep onset delay. *Journal of autism and developmental disorders., 45*(1), 100 - 110.

Warrier, V. G. (2020). Elevated rates of autism, other neurodevelopmental and psychiatric diagnoses, and autistic traits in transgender and gender-diverse individuals. *Nature Communications.*

Weiss, J. A. (2018). Victimization and Perpetration Experiences of Adults With Autism. *Frontiers in psychiatry*, 203.

Woods, R. (2020). Pathological Demand Avoidance (PDA). In F. Volkmar, *Encyclopedia of Autism Spectrum Disorders.* New York: Springer.

Yeager, K. &.-W. (2013). Cultural humility: Essential foundation for clinical researchers. *Applied Nursing Research*, 251-256.

APPENDIX A

Questions to ask potential therapists include:

1. How and/or where did you learn about autism?

- Ideally the practitioner will have engaged in learning beyond their formal education, which is often grounded in the medical model, and lacking in high quality autism specific content. Learning may take the form of Continuing Professional Development (CPD), or self-directed study. Learning from folk with lived experience is important.

2. Can you tell me a little bit about your experience working with autistic clients?

- Inexperience is not always a negative, but it is usually more helpful to work with a practitioner who has some experience working with autistic clients and understands our unique needs.

3. How would you describe Autism?

- Listen for pathologising language and affirming language. Choose a practitioner who uses affirming language.

4. Are you familiar with neurodiversity affirming practices?

• Ideally the answer will be a firm yes.

5. Would you consider your approach neurodiversity affirming? If so, how so?

• Again, the ideal answer is a firm yes. A neurodiversity affirming approach is grounded in the social model of disability, rejects ableist perspectives on autism, is person-centred, and promotes self-advocacy.

6. What are the main therapeutic approaches you use (e.g., CBT)

• There is no right or wrong here, however many modalities have been adapted to suit neurodivergent folk. It is most important that the practitioners approach is person-centred.

7. Do you have experience working with (your specific area of concern)?

• Relevant experience, while not essential, is usually helpful.

8. Do you offer remote sessions (i.e., via phone or video)?

• Remote access will be very important for some, less so for others. It is up to you to decide whether this is something you want or need.

9. Is your practice an autism-friendly environment?

- An autism friendly environment is one that welcomes you to come as you are, invites you to unmask, and makes every effort to accommodate your individual differences and needs. Not all practices will have sensory tools and other supports available, but many will, and those that do not would ideally invite you to bring your own.

10. Do you identify as neurodivergent yourself?

- I debated whether to include this question as I know many exceptional neurotypical therapists who work beautifully with neurodivergent clients, and I do not wish to confuse readers by suggesting that lived experience is a requirement for therapists working with neurodivergent folk. It is not. Also, one's neurotype is private information, and deciding not to disclose it to clients (or anyone, for that matter) is a perfectly reasonable choice. That said, I understand it is important to some people to know whether the professionals on their team belong to the neurodivergent community, and I also believe that the therapeutic alliance tends to be strengthened by transparency. The invitation is to use your own judgement when deciding if, and when, to ask this question. If the answer is important to you, go ahead and ask, and be open to the possibility that the practitioner may exercise their right to respectfully decline to answer.

www.ingramcontent.com/pod-product-compliance
Lightning Source LLC
Chambersburg PA
CBHW060505280326
41933CB00014B/2867